CINEMA EAST

CINEMA EAST

A Critical Study
of Major Japanese Films

Keiko I. McDonald

RUTHERFORD ● MADISON ● TEANECK
FAIRLEIGH DICKINSON UNIVERSITY PRESS
LONDON AND TORONTO: ASSOCIATED UNIVERSITY PRESSES

Associated University Presses, Inc.
4 Cornwall Drive
East Brunswick, N.J. 08816

Associated University Presses Ltd
27 Chancery Lane
London WC2A 1NF, England

Associated University Presses
2133 Royal Windsor Drive
Unit 1
Mississauga, Ontario
Canada L5J 1K5

Library of Congress Cataloging in Publication Data

McDonald, Keiko I.
    Cinema East.

    Bibliography: p.
    1. Moving-pictures—Japan.   2. Moving-picture plays
—History and criticism.   I. Title.
PN1993.5.J3M35   1983   791.43'0952   81-65870
ISBN 0-8386-3094-4

Printed in the United States of America

To Donald Richie

Contents

Acknowledgments

The writing of this book was made possible by the generous assistance of a number of people, to all of whom I am very grateful.

I would like to express my sincerest gratitude to my mentor, Donald Richie, international authority on Japanese cinema, who unselfishly devoted his time to offering me as much professional assistance as possible. Without his generous help and warm encouragement, this book would never have been completed.

I also owe a great debt of gratitude to Douglas Umstead, chairman of the Department of Romance Languages at Kent State University, whose constructive criticism of my manuscript helped to make this book more substantial.

I would also like to offer special thanks to Tadao Satō, a foremost film critic of Japan, for offering me valuable information on films by Kurosawa and Mizoguchi.

I am very grateful to William Cadbury from the Department of English of the University of Oregon for offering a series of inspiring lectures, which helped me to form the critical framework of this book.

I am also greatly indebted to Howard Boksenbaum and Jan-Paul Malocsay, who went over my manuscript and made useful suggestions from the viewpoint of the American audience.

I would like to thank Kazuo Miyagawa, a director of photography of international renown, who provided me with useful information on *Rashomon*, *Ugetsu*, and *The Key*, for which he was the director of photography.

Akira Shimizu from the Japan Library Film Council, Sadamu Maruo and Masatoshi Ōba from the Film Center of the Tokyo National Museum of Modern Art, and Charles Silber from the Film Center of the New York Museum of Modern Art kindly helped my research by arranging private screenings of a great number of films.

Research work for this book, which took me to Japan for the three consecutive summers of 1976, 1977, and 1978, was supported in part by a Fulbright-Hays grant from the U.S. Office of Education, a grant from the National Endowment for the Humanities, a summer grant from the University of Pittsburgh, and a faculty research grant from the Japan Iron and Steel Federation Endowment Fund of the University of Pittsburgh. I owe a special debt of thanks to these organizations as well.

Introduction: A Search for Unity

As early as 1951, Kurosawa's *Rashomon*, the Grand Prize winner at the Venice Festival, awakened the international film audience to the merits of Japanese cinema. Since then, a great many Japanese films have come to be known throughout the world as cinema classics.

The number of Japanese film masterpieces dating from the 1950s has prompted some critics to say that the decade marks the maturity of sound films in Japan, in contrast to the so-called golden age of Japanese silent films in the 1930s. Most Japanese cinematic masters entered the decade already fairly well established. They included directors like Kenji Mizoguchi, Yasujirō Ozu, Mikio Naruse, Keisuke Kinoshita, Tadashi Imai, Kon Ichikawa, and Akira Kurosawa. The films of these directors in this period exhibit a breadth and confidence that brings a kind of maturity to themes, which, in many cases, had occupied them in the late 1940s after World War II and/or even before it.

Many critics still consider it "too soon to determine if the 1960s are the last golden age of Japanese cinema."[1] But a goodly number of new names arrived on the "New Wave," as it was called, because of elements of experiment and controversy that are reminiscent of the French *nouvelle vague*. Notable among the talented young directors of the 1960s are Nagisa Ōshima, Masahiro Shinoda, Yoshishige Yoshida, Hiroshi Teshigahara, Shōhei Imamura, and Kinji Fukasaku. Confrontation may be the keynote here, since these directors used bold new techniques and themes related to new problems confronting postwar Japanese society. Teshigahara, for example, posed existential questions; Kinji Fukasaku brought a new note of violence to the Yakuza genre film; and Ōshima explored political issues in dynamic ways, even as he also experimented with situations of Brechtian estrangement. Shinoda and Yoshida studied love and violence, making use of novel aesthetic points of view. Imamura pursued the subject of primitivism in modern Japan: incest, patriarchy, and so forth.

11

A glance at a standard survey—*Nihon Eiga Hyakusen* [*One Hundred Selections of Japanese Cinema*] by Tadao Satō and Kyōichirō Nanbu—shows how secure a place these directors hold in the development of postwar Japanese cinema.[2] Take, for example, Ozu, whom many of his countrymen consider "the most Japanese of all their directors."[3] During this period, Ozu directed films that present his traditional treatment of middle-class family life: *Early Summer* [Bakushū, 1951]; *Tokyo Story* [Tokyo Monogatari, 1953]; and *Equinox Flower* [Higanbana, 1958]. Mizoguchi enjoys high praise for his three international prizewinners: *The Life of Oharu* [Saikaku Ichidai Onna, 1952]; *Ugetsu* [Ugetsu Monogatari, 1953]; and *The Crucified Lovers* [Chikamatsu Monogatari, 1954]. The films by Kurosawa included are *Ikiru* (1953); *Seven Samurai* [Shichinin no Samurai, 1954]; and *Rashomon* (1950). Imai's melodrama, *Until the Day We Meet Again* [Mata Au Hi Made, 1950], along with his social drama, *Darkness at Noon* [Mahiru no Ankoku, 1956], adds a new generic dimension to the list. Kinoshita also makes a valuable contribution to the selection with his *Carmen Comes Home* [Karumen Kokyō ni Kaeru,, 1951]; *You Were like a Wild Chrysanthemum* [Nogiku no Gotoki Kimi Nariki, 1955]; *The Ballad of the Naruyama* [Naruyamabushi-kō, 1958]; and *Twenty-four Eyes* [Nijūshi no Hitomi, 1954], cited as "the most tear-jerking film in the history of Japanese cinema.

Kon Ichikawa's representative films, *Fire on the Plain* [Nobi, 1959] and *Younger Brother* [Otōto, 1960] are also included among the best one hundred Japanese films. Ōshima, a leading figure in the Japanese *nouvelle vague* movement, enjoys a lion's share of attention with *Night and Fog in Japan* [Nihon no Yoru to Kiri, 1960]; *A Cruel Story of Youth* [Seishun Zankoku Monogatari, 1960]; *Death by Hanging* [Kōshikei, 1968]; and *Boy* [Shōnen, 1969]. Shinoda, another important figure in the movement, receives sound critical attention from Satō and Nanbu for his *Double Suicide* [Shinjū Ten no Amijima, 1969] and *Assassination* [Ansatsu, 1964]. The 1965 Cannes Festival First Prize winner, *The Woman in the Dunes* [Suna no Onna, 1964] by Hiroshi Teshigahara, also receives its fair share of recognition. Mikio Naruse is represented by *Lightning* [Inazuma, 1952] and *Floating Clouds* [Ukigumo, 1955], and Shōhei Imamura by *Pigs and Battleship* [Buta to Gunkan, 1961]; *The Insect Woman* [Nippon Konchūki, 1963]; *Intentions of Murder* [Akai Satsui, 1964]; and *The Profound Desire of the Gods* [Kamigami no Fukaki Yokubō, 1968]. Satō and Nanbu also include in their selection Yoshida's *Eros plus Massacre* [Erosu Purasu Gyakusatsu, 1969].

A number of books have been written to serve the growing Western audience for Japanese cinema. The first really authoritative survey of Japanese cinema in English is *The Japanese Film: Art and Industry* (1960) by Joseph Anderson and Donald Richie. Another important work is *The Japanese Movie: An Illustrated History* (1966), by Donald Richie, which offers an illuminating account of the development of Japanese cinema from 1896 on. Richie's more recent book, *Japanese Cinema: Film Style and National Character* (1971), complements his treatment of the films with a combination of contextual, historical, and aesthetic approaches, and offers a broad, yet critical survey of directors in terms of their cinematic techniques, thematic concerns, and contributions to Japanese film history. Another recent book, Richard Tucker's *Japan: Film Image* (1973) provides a rather sketchy chronological survey of leading Japanese directors and representative works.

In the early 1970s, the critical works focused on particular directors like Kurosawa and Ozu. Among these is Paul Schrader's crosscultural study, *Transcendental Style in Film: Ozu, Bresson, Dreyer* (1972). *Focus on Rashomon* (1972), edited by Richie, contains a collection of critical essays (his own included). One of Richie's other works, *The Films of Akira Kurosawa* (1970), is devoted to intensive analyses of films from historical contextual and technical viewpoints. Richie has also recently published *Ozu: His Life and Films* (1974), a critical examination of scripts, shooting, and editing of that director's entire output.

Since the mid-1970s, a number of books have appeared in response to the rapid shifting critical orientations in film studies. A few of these works offer stronger organizational principles and/or even ideological commitments. Among these are two works by Joan Mellen. *Voices from the Japanese Cinema* (1975) is a collection of interviews with major directors, with emphasis on their ideologies and ambitions. *The Waves at Genji's Door: Japan Through Its Cinema* is a view of the Japanese social and cultural milieu from various vantage points with special attention to feminist perspectives seen through films.

In his recent book, *To the Distant Observer: Form and Meaning in the Japanese Cinema* (1979), Noël Burch applies a unique critical method to a larger number of Japanese films, some made before World War II. His insistence on a combination of Marxist/semioticist perspectives leads to an emphasis on form at the expense of content and sometimes to a misinterpretation of issues in films. Burch, however, does provide many cogent observations, especially on formal aspects of various films.

Audie Bock's *Japanese Film Directors* (1979) offers an orthodox

historical approach to leading Japanese filmmakers. Though each
chapter of this book contains a fairly detailed discussion of one
representative work by each director, Bock's criticism focuses on
the times closely connected with the production of those works.

Even a cursory glance at criticism in English of Japanese cinema
shows that much remains to be done; it shows a need for an in-
depth study of individual Japanese films. I have two reasons for
offering this series of studies of great Japanese films from the 1950s
and 1960s.

First and foremost, my experience in teaching Japanese film
courses to American students has put me in direct contact with the
basic question: "How does one *show* Western viewers, primarily
general audiences, how to *see* a Japanese film?" I hope that this book
offers some answers to that question.

My second reason is more personal, since the study of Japanese
cinema in the United States involves questions of cultural differences and—for a Japanese person like myself—it involves questions
of cultural identity as well. Even though other Japanese film critics
will not necessarily agree with my readings of these films, most
would probably agree that one of the best ways to test one's understanding of one's own culture is to introduce someone else to it. Of
course, that is done, at best, obliquely in criticism confined to
single films; but again, I hope that these brief studies of Japanese
films will at least introduce the audience to the need to study crosscultural perspectives.

It goes without saying that Japanese films of the 1950s and 1960s
offer an embarrassment of riches from which to choose. Still, it is
the critic's pleasure to comment on works that suit his or her
methods and interests. Another principle of selection is purely mechanical. So many important Japanese films are simply not yet
available in the United States.[4]

My methods are primarily those of the literary critic who considers each film as a finished product (rather than one "in process"),
an organic whole, a self-contained entity.

Naturally, such a critic begins with questions of structure. As
with any literary work, a film may be viewed from two perspectives: internal and external. The former confines itself to what
happens *in* the film, with its parts and how they relate to one
another. For example, the internal perspective studies individual
characters in relation to the world and the problems they confront,
and their subsequent attempts at solutions. Viewed "internally," a
film may be seen to represent life realistically, or not; and charac-

ters may be viewed as individuals or as types. These types may represent some larger entity, such as a system of values, or superheroes expressive of our self-identity fantasies.

Symbols may serve internal functions as important as those served by the characters themselves. In film studies influenced by structuralism and semiotics, the term *symbol* has become rather ambiguous. In my analyses I follow James Monaco in defining *symbol* as "something that represents something else by resemblance, association, or convention."

Mood, or atmosphere, is another basic internal element, and is a speciality of directors like Mizoguchi and Ozu. The Japanese are notoriously sensitive to the way the outside world evokes, or corresponds to, inner states of being. For this reason, as Donald Richie notes, the merging of individual characters with their surroundings is a characteristic device of Japanese film directors—one that says important things about their use of space.[5]

Similarly, such elements as time, spatial differentiation, and story function internally.

Like any literary work, a film marshals its effects in order to clarify the central problem, which is expressed through a protagonist's manner of relating to his or her world and the choices it invites or forces the protagonist to make. Some options may seem mutually exclusive, others may seem uneasily compatible, and still others may seem "free," a matter of roads taken, or not taken. In any case, the protagonist's behavior offers us important clues to the world view at work—whether it is to be taken as tragic, or comic, or romantic, or ironic.

The other perspective, the external one on the structure of a film, invites us to relate all these elements to the audience. It entails the protagonist's feelings, degree of involvement, and notion of good or bad as related to characters, action, and value.[6] There is a lot to say about the way Japanese directors manipulate audience response, making of it something not less than an integral part of the structure of some films. Put another way, we might say that the art of cinema is especially intimate with its beholder. We see this when we study questions of interpretation of a protagonist's behavior. We ask whether we are being asked to take up an attitude of simple identification with, or rejection of, the given protagonist or outcome. Or as we shall see, a director may offer, or even, enforce, more complex responses: he may refuse to tell us clearly what to "do."

Of course, devices of internal/external structure are inseparably united through the use of the third basic of cinematic art: camera technique. This is discussed separately in each chapter in order to clarify aspects of a given director's style, and to show how the director's use of the camera provides important clues to his intentions.

Mizoguchi, for example, prefers the one-scene-one-shot method, with vigorous panning and dollying as well, though notably sparing of the close-up. By "reading" his intentions through his camera work, we can see how Mizoguchi means, for example, to intensify our sense of a character's response to a given environment by emphasizing *it*. Moreover, the camera also shows us how the director himself wants to project his own feelings about the character onto the scene.

Similarly, we see Ozu preferring three standard shots: the long, medium, and close-up—this last being used to study moments of heightened emotion.[7] This might appear to be a more intimate approach, yet we must also take into account Ozu's formalistic tendency, which puts the audience at a certain distance from the characters who are studied closely.

Kurosawa's photography, to choose one more example, is characteristically low-key in some films. This is aimed at creating a gloomy atmosphere expressive of a desire to objectify psychological states or the underlying causes of fragmented societies.

An interesting characteristic of the younger directors of the *nouvelle vague* of the 1960s is an extremely mobile camera. Here we see more than one director using the camera itself to discourage any tendency the viewer may have to take a rigid, complacent, or even cinematically "final" view of the matter at hand. Here we see directors proposing a relationship of notable uneasiness as they ask us to share their interest in questions with, possibly, no answers.

A film must, of course, solve the aesthetic problems it sets itself, and does this by reconciling its internal and external structure through the camera. To explain how this is done requires detailed rehearsal of scenes and sequences that some readers may find trying. This is especially true with two films: *Death by Hanging* and *Eros plus Massacre*, both of which are highly complex in their method of presentation and use of verbal interplay. The reader who studies the concept of a given film this way, however, stands a much better chance of seeing *into* the complex masterpieces of the art that make their ways across seas and cultures so remote from the land of their origins.

NOTES

1. Audie Bock, *Japanese Film Directors* (Tokyo: Kōdansha International, 1978), p. 14.

2. Tadao Satō and Kyōichirō Nanbu, *Nihon Eiga Hyakusen* [One Hundred Selections of Japanese Cinema] (Tokyo: Akita Shoten, 1973). Their selection criteria are purely thematic and rhetorical: they have chosen the one hundred films that best present vivid images of individuals living different kinds of lives and best provide a perspective on life that most viewers are unlikely to have experienced. See Preface.

3. Donald Richie, *Ozu: His Life and Films* (Berkeley: University of California Press, 1974), p. xi.

4. One such is Shindō's *The Iron Crown* [Kanawa, 1971]. Its use of time sequence is extremely ingenious. I have, however, been able to discuss Yoshida's *Eros plus Massacre*, which is currently available only with French subtitles. However, acknowledging that the film, a recent great work, is worth analyzing, and also assuming that it will soon be released with English subtitles, I have included it here. Among the Japanese films produced in the 1960s, *Eros plus Massacre* is cited as one of the most difficult ones. Therefore, I have tried to be much more descriptive of the film's action than I was in my discussion of the other films. Naruse's *Floating Clouds* articulates the typical Naruse mood pertinent to the particular world view of the postwar period, as revealed in the seamy aspects of love between man and woman. However, I have purposely eliminated this film because I have learned that it has been released in the U.S. only recently and that Audie Bock's forthcoming dissertation studies Naruse's films.

5. Donald Richie, *Japanese Cinema: Film Style and National Character* (Garden City, N.Y.: Doubleday Anchor, 1971), pp. xix–xx.

6. William Cadbury's article, "Character and the Mock Heroic in *Barchester Towers*," provides a detailed treatment of different points of view taken by the reader in order to achieve a coherent vision of the novel. See *Texas Studies in Literature and Language* 5 (1963): 569.

7. For a fuller treatment of Ozu's basic shots, see Donald Richie, "Yasujiro Ozu: The Syntax of His Films," *Film Quarterly* 18 (Winter 1963–1964): 11–16.

CINEMA
EAST

Part 1
SYMBOLISM

1

The Dialectic of Light and Darkness in Kurosawa's *Rashomon*

Akira Kurosawa's *Rashomon*, the winner of both the 1951 Venice Festival Grand Prize and the 1952 Academy Award for Best Foreign Film, has been examined from many perspectives. One Japanese critic has pointed to the non-Japanese qualities of *Rashomon* and Kurosawa's other major films,[1] and another critic has commented on its fine filmic style.[2] A number of Western critics have explored the moral, psychological, and social implications of the murder in the film and its consequence.[3] When he was once asked what *Rashomon* is about, Kurosawa simply stated that the film is about rape and nothing more. This statement by Kurosawa encourages us to interpret the film in any possible way that will satisfy our critical propensity. No critic has yet approached *Rashomon* from the vantage point of symbolism, even though this perspective offers a key insight into the central problem of this difficult film: "What is man's nature?"

Rashomon is pervaded by a dialectic of symbols of light and darkness. The murder takes place in a dense, dark forest. The main actions of the priest, the woodcutter, and the commoner are set against the pouring rain. The half-ruined gate standing in the torrent gives the film a gloomy setting. In sharp contrast to these dark images are impressionistically filmed images of sunlight. The blazing sun piercing the clouds dominates the police station. Sunlight coming through the trees flickers on the woodcutter's ax. When the wife yields to the bandit, she looks up at the sun glittering through the branches. At the conclusion of the film the woodcutter walks into the sunlight after the rainstorm is over. The juxtaposition of these symbols serves as an important, basic constituent, which contributes to a unified vision of the film.

Rashomon opens with ten rapid shots of a half-ruined gate, the Rashomon, in the midst of a downpour. These shots are followed by the subtitle, which reads: "Kyoto, in the twelfth century when famines and civil wars had devastated the ancient capital." In the following scene the gloom these natural and man-made calamities connote is intensified by the priest's remark: "Wars, earthquakes, great winds, fires, famines, plague—each new year is full of disaster." So it was in the twelfth century, which marked Japan's transition from aristocracy to feudalism; it was a period characterized by political turmoil.[4] Buddhist religious thinkers of that century believed that they were witnessing the final degenerate phase of the world, which would soon end in apocalypse. Disasters like those mentioned by the priest were taken as signs of the world's approaching end.[5]

It is thus clear why the movie starts with a keen awareness of the fragmented state of the world. Both the ruined state of the Rashomon gate, once the splendid southern entrance to the capital, and the violent rain symbolize the chaos prevailing in the world. Yet, two major components of the gate—the gargoyle and the signboard—appear intact amid the devastation. The integrity of these two religious symbols implies that religion has not been completely destroyed but, in fact, holds out a potential for the restoration of order.

Immediately after the second close-up of the signboard, which bears the characters, "Rashomon," the woodcutter begins to recount his discovery of the murdered samurai. A flashback swiftly takes the viewer to the forest where the murder took place. When the woodcutter's story ends, the dark forest suddenly yields to the sunlit police station where the priest, the woodcutter, the wife, and the thief are brought out. First, the priest offers his version of what happened. Then the thief, Tajōmaru, provides his version of the story, which we are shown taking place in the forest. When the thief finishes his story, the forest suddenly vanishes as we return first to the police station, and then swiftly again to the half-ruined Rashomon gate. This same pattern of transitions is repeated as the wife tells her version of the story, and the husband his. The tight architectonics of the flashback is important for three reasons. First, each time the scene is cut back to the gate where the film started, the debate over man's nature between the priest and the commoner becomes more intense. Second, the flashback molds Kurosawa's basic design of the dual symbolism: from the darkness of the forest to the light of the police station and back again to the darkness in the gate. Third, the three repetitive geographical changes make a smooth transition to the woodcutter's nature that has occupied the priest and the commoner.

When Tajōmaru has explained how the rape took place, the commoner, the woodcutter, and the priest start discussing the reliability of his testimony. The woodcutter simply states that Tajōmaru's confession is "a lie." By so doing, the woodcutter functions as an instigator increasing the intensity of argument between the priest and the commoner, who explain their own reasons for rejecting Tajōmaru's version. Both the commoner and the priest agree that man is by nature a liar. However, this very agreement reveals their radically different perspectives on human nature. The commoner is realistic; he assumes that man is innately an impulsive and selfish creature. He further claims that it is thus impossible to avoid lies especially in difficult times like the present. On the other hand, the priest is idealistic; he assumes that man is basically a rational creature. He argues that deception is a part of an illusion that man cultivates as a necessary tool in confronting the hostile reality of life. The two scenes at the gate, which respectively follow the woman's and the husband's (through the medium's mouth) narrations, clarify these two antithetical perspectives on man's nature. In response to the woodcutter's insistence that their stories are equally untruthful, the priest says: "I must not believe that men are so sinful." Conversely, the commoner says: "After all, who's honest nowadays? Look, everyone wants to forget unpleasant things, so they make up stories."

From this discussion, the central problem of the film is evident: "Is man's nature essentially rational or impulsive, good or bad?" The film presents three basic answers in response. A rationalistic answer is presented by the priest, a primitivistic answer is represented by the commoner, and a melioristic response emerges in the final part of the film. This final answer, given through the woodcutter, is a synthesis of the previous two stances. It claims that man's character includes a separation between reason and impulse, but that man is good to the extent that he tries to reduce this separation. From this perspective, the different versions of the murder in the forest can be taken all together as an answer to the central problem. Kurosawa seems to say we must probe the question of man's nature by playing the various accounts of the murder against one another. The existence of the conflicting stories implies that if man is put through the ordeal of life, the way he acts will reveal his inner nature.

This philosophic concern with man's inner nature as revealed through his behavior is also a feature of Kurosawa's samurai films, such as *The Throne of Blood* and *Seven Samurai*. In *The Throne of Blood*, Washizu, the Japanese Macbeth, swept by his "bolting ambition" into the turmoil of civil war, is trapped in an intellectual maze that causes his destruction. The seven samurai are initially motivated by a desire to satisfy their hunger and agree to help the seemingly hopeless farmers; however, through their battles with bandits, the Samurai gradually become altruists. It is not their words but their actions that illuminate the Samurais' inner nature. The theme of the revelation of man's inner reality is also explored in such naturalistic novels as Joseph Conrad's *Heart of Darkness*, which evolves around a man's metaphysical journey into the depths of his heart. These films and literary works present man as a combination of an outer self and an inner self: the outer self, donning a social mask, is controlled by reason that affiliates itself with existing ethical norms; on the other hand, the inner self is controlled by impulses.

The implications of light and darkness are rather opaque in *Rashomon*. On one level, the dichotomy of light and darkness, then, can be considered as an archetypical representation of this bifurcation of man's nature: light represents reason whereas darkness represents impulse. Significantly, darkness is treated as negative until the final sequence of the film because Kurosawa presents impulses as deviations from man's moral consciousness. Then, at the second level, light represents good in man whereas darkness represents evil.

When the woodcutter goes into the dark woods at the beginning of *Rashomon*, the sun is flickering on his ax through the bushes. This glinting sun, which most critics cite as a prime example of Kurosawa's impressionism,[6] symbolizes the exertion of man's moral consciousness over his impulsive action. As the woodcutter continues on into the forest, the sky is again visible through the branches of the trees overhead. The repeated juxtaposition of light and darkness keeps reminding the viewer of the bifurcation of man's nature. The woodcutter first finds a woman's hat with a veil on a branch of a tree. Then he finds a man's hat at his feet, and then a piece of rope. Finally he comes upon an amulet case lying on the leaves. Kurosawa films these objects all in close-up, calling our attention to their symbolic significance. The hats are important social symbols of the station of the samurai and his wife. The amulet case represents man's adherence to religion. Combined with the sense of liberation implied by the torn tope, the abandoned social adornments symbolize the elimination of layers of the social mask, hence, the outer self.

Thus, what happened to the woodcutter, the samurai, his wife, and the thief in the forest is, on a symbolic level, a centripetal regression into the inner self. The apparently incongruous stories given by these four, however, lead us to believe that each person's self-image is radically different from the image he conveys to the others. The woodcutter confesses that he has not seen the dagger that penetrated the husband's chest, and therefore, he is innocent of its theft. The commoner claims, however, that there is good reason to believe that the woodcutter stole the dagger. Although the wife, Masago, insists that she was raped, the stories given by her husband and Tajōmaru affirm that she enjoyed the sexual encounter. The woodcutter's story and Masago's describe the husband as lacking in physical strength and being devoid of compassion. On the contrary, the husband's version asserts that he was true to the samurai code. In his confession, Tajōmaru stresses his bravery and skill at swordsmanship. However, in the woodcutter's story, the duel between Tajōmaru and the samurai, in which they "crossed swords over twenty times" is the very antithesis of the ideal samurai duel. Tajōmaru is described as an equal match only because the samurai is a weak, poor swordsman.

Assimilating the stories related by these four characters, we can make a reasonable deduction that each character succumbed to his inner nature in a precarious situation. The woodcutter, a victim of his greed, loses the power to curb his urge to steal the dagger. The film's visual action presents the woodcutter flabbergasted, dropping his glittering ax upon encountering the samurai's corpse. This gesture externalizes his loss of control.

Likewise, Masago yielded to passion though initially reason tried to suppress her impulse. Kurosawa elaborately cinematizes her moral dilemma through the juxtaposition of light and darkness. When the bandit starts kissing her, she looks straight up into the sunlight. The swift crosscutting between Masago staring up at the sun and the dazzling sunlight penetrating the branches culminates in a slow fade-out of the sun. The fade-out is immediately succeeded by a close-up of Masago closing her eyes—a gesture emblematic of her loss of reason. As she lets go of her outer nature, Masago lets go of her dagger, the means of protection that a samurai's wife characteristically carried. The camera slowly tracks up toward Tajōmaru and Masago, and catches her fingers in a medium shot as her grip on Tajōmaru becomes gradually tighter.

In the depths of the forest, the samurai has disclosed his fear, cowardice, and selfishness, completely contrary to his outwardly stern *bushido* nature. As described by the woodcutter, when the samurai frees himself from the rope, he tells Tajōmaru, nervously retreating from the bandit: "Stop! I refuse to risk my life for such a woman." Rather than protecting his wife from the bandit, the Samurai tries to protect himself. When the samurai and the bandit eventually do start to fight after Masago's provocative remarks that both of them should prove themselves to be real men by fighting, the samurai's action betrays his weakness and ineptitude. Kurosawa's camera work helps to visualize the samurai's cowardice. By persistently employing a medium shot deploying both the samurai and Tajōmaru along an almost horizontal line, Kurosawa emphasizes not only the samurai's consciousness of Tajōmaru as an equal match but also his timorousness. Another device used by Kurosawa is the frequent presentation of the samurai's physiognomy in a medium shot. This is an effective device for drawing our attention to the samurai's emotion even as it keeps us from becoming too much involved in it. For example, when the samurai slowly advances toward Tajōmaru, the medium shot of the samurai's face reveals terror. Consequently, as we expected, he fails to meet the opponent's challenge as a samurai and screams: "I don't want to die! I don't want to die!"

More surprisingly, Tajōmaru, whom the commoner describes as "worse than all the other bandits in Kyoto" has yielded to cowardice in the forest. During the battle, as narrated by the woodcutter, Kurosawa pervasively resorts to a medium shot of Tajōmaru's face full of his fear and anxiety. Kurosawa also takes care in the visual alignment of Tajōmaru and the samurai. In Tajōmaru's own story, Kurosawa lets the bandit's back dominate the screen while placing the samurai at the further end. Conversely, in the woodcutter's version, a medium shot of Tajōmaru and the samurai aligned on a horizontal line across the screen forms the basic composition. This ironic contrast plays down the bandit's powerfulness and conveys to us the emptiness of his bravado. Consequently, when the samurai advances, Tajōmaru's arms start shaking violently. Tajōmaru approaches the samurai slowly and fearfully. Finally, when Masago runs into the woods, Tajōmaru collapses on the ground.

Exposed to the sunlight at the police station, the woodcutter, the samurai, Masago, and Tajōmaru all tell their stories, faithful to their own illusions of what they should be. The sunlight over their heads symbolizes their return to reason. They don their social masks and confess in a manner that will protect their self-images and justify their actions. In contrast to the earlier scenes of the forest, the police station scene is dominated by Kurosawa's more restrictive camera movement and visual composition. The priest, the woodcutter, the wife, and the bandit all sit in a line across the screen, and they are shot from the eye level of the policeman taking their testimony.[7] The camera angle elevates us to the position of the police, the objective judge. The fact that each person is avoiding the eyes of the camera as if afraid of the judgment encourages us to search below the surface in order to distinguish reality from appearance. Interestingly, in the forest scenes Kurosawa pervasively used the point-of-view shot to emphasize each narrator's view of the others involved in the murder. However, the shift in his camera work does not necessarily correspond to the shift in our perspective from identification to detachment. Rather, this change in the camera work augments our sense of detachment, i.e., outside view, which is necessary for a coherent reading of the film.

At this stage the conflicting narrations may yield a tentative acceptance of the commoner's view of man's nature; man is an impulsive creature when confronted with the fragmented world. However, the final interaction of the woodcutter, the priest, and the commoner not only clarifies the three views of man's nature more fully but also asserts the stance represented by the woodcutter. When the woodcutter's second story finally ends the series of stories, Kurosawa brings us back to the Rashomon gate, to the realist and idealist, the commoner and the priest. It is still raining. The commoner says: "The world we live in is a hell." None of the testimony has moved him an inch from his "realistic" view of human existence as a matter of dog-eat-dog. As if to emphasize the point, the commoner starts tearing wood off the sacred gate to make a fire, and steals the foundling's clothes. Significantly the commoner's attire itself symbolically affirms his stance. At the beginning of the film, he takes off his shirt and is filmed half-naked, that is, without his social mask.

Similarly, the priest reasserts his idealistic view that man is capable of good; that even when man lies, he lies through recourse to reason, even if it is a purely selfish reason like self-defense. The priest prefers rational moral bad choices to chaotic impulsive violence. The priest's decent robes symbolically correspond to the stance that man assumes many layers of social disguise.

With the introduction of the image of the baby, the film's action takes a radical turn. It moves from the static to the dynamic. Turning away from their debate over man's nature, the priest, the commoner, and the woodcutter now act out their respective views. The subsequent scenes mark the beginning of the final answer to the hitherto sustained central problem. When the commoner sees the baby, his reaction is to kneel over it and strip it of its clothes. The commoner acts out his view that man is impulsive. At the same time his action is presented as negative because the baby is a symbol of fertility and future, and the theft of its clothes constitutes the extermination of hope for a better society. On the other hand, both the priest and the woodcutter respond to the situation rationally. They rush toward the baby, whom the priest holds protectively. The woodcutter, who has been verbally inexpressive of his own view of man's nature, now shows his opinion through action; he tries to support the priest's view and defend goodness, which he thinks still remains within man. The woodcutter accuses the commoner of being evil and selfish, and calls his conduct atrocious.

Earlier Kurosawa introduced the abandoned amulet case, but this time he introduces an amulet case fastened to the baby. This amulet case makes us aware of the possibility of future religious salvation in this fragmented world. In response to the woodcutter's accusation, the commoner says: "And what's wrong with it? That's the way we are, the way we live. Look, half of us envy the lives that dogs lead. You just can't live unless you're what you call selfish."

The subsequent cinematic action portrays a struggle between the woodcutter and the commoner in the rain. The scene is symbolically crucial in that it externalizes the tension between the primitivism asserted by the commoner and the rationalism asserted by the priest and now tentatively assumed by the woodcutter. The destructive rain, in which the battle is set, symbolizes the social milieu that places these two metaphysical positions in conflict. Their battle ends when the commoner accuses the woodcutter of stealing the dagger. The woodcutter's defense of the priest's rationalism thus quickly gives way to the commoner's primitivism. The woodcutter says: "All men are selfish and dishonest." Yet, unlike the commoner, the woodcutter tries to justify man's inclination toward primitivism on the ground of social determinism. He says: "They all have excuses, the bandit, the husband . . ." Deeply affected by the commoner's statement that he "may have fooled the police," the woodcutter's conviction that man is rational and good has now become totally shaken.

In order to dramatize the ascendancy of primitivism over rationalism, which ensues from the conflict between the woodcutter and the commoner, Kurosawa plays upon contrasting physiognomy: the commoner's triumphant, smiling face and the woodcutter's sad, guilty face, both taken in close-up. The commoner continues to push the woodcutter toward the priest, who has been watching the struggle between the two. The commoner's accusation continues: "And so where is that dagger? Did the earth open up and swallow it? Or did someone steal it? Am I right? It would seem so. Now there is a really selfish action for you." Kurosawa swiftly cuts from a medium shot of the commoner slapping the woodcutter to a close-up of the priest holding the baby.

The following long shot, which is focused on the three men under the half-ruined gate, once again imposes a distancing effect upon us, and encourages us to contemplate the three possible views of man's nature. The commoner disappears into the rain, leaving the other two under the gate. By associating the commoner with the torrent, Kurosawa seems to equate the primitive with the destructive side of man's nature and thus to discourage us from accepting this view. The next long shot shows the half-ruined gate, looming above the two men who seem extremely small, intensifying the sense of man's hopelessness in coping with environmental forces.

The three shots following the commoner's disappearance into the rain are thematically significant in three respects. First, these shots, each terminated by a dissolve, mark a radical transition from darkness to light. Second, the dialectic of the two perspectives on man's nature now assumed by the woodcutter and the priest is kept in a tension that will later yield to resolution. A long shot of the priest and the commoner standing under the gate is quickly taken over by a medium shot of both men. At precisely this moment the sound of the rain ceases. Another medium shot of the two remains to be presented while the raindrops thin. Next, a close-up of the priest and the woodcutter under the gate is projected, and the silence is suddenly broken by the baby's cry. The rhetorical stance imposed upon the audience is detachment, since the succession of the simultaneous shots of these two men keeps the audience from identifying with either of them. Again Kurosawa visualizes the polar views through physiognomy; whereas the priest's face is almost impassive, the woodcutter's face is full of remorse, guilt, and compassion.

Referring to the dissolve, which terminates each of the three shots, Donald Richie states that this technique usually means time passing, that it is at the same time a formal gesture, "a gesture which makes us look, makes us feel."[8] Thus, the final important function of the three shots is that the dissolve emphasizes the lapse of psychological time during which the woodcutter's mind goes through a radical transformation—a transformation which might have escaped the audience's attention had a simple cut been used. The guilt and remorse over what the woodcutter did in the forest awaken compassion for the foundling. Precisely at this juncture, reason and impulse join in harmony in his mind. Compassion, a most important Buddhist principle, becomes the root of his moral consciousness: it is what society would have him act upon. The transition from rain into sunlight clearly corresponds to the woodcutter's psychological change.

The following scene reveals that the priest's hitherto unshaken assumption that man is rational and benign has been somewhat affected by what he has thus far witnessed. When the woodcutter tries to take the baby, the priest recoils. The woodcutter humbly responds: "I have six children of my own. One more wouldn't make it any more difficult." The priest apologizes for having suspected the woodcutter's motive: "No. I'm grateful to you. Because, thanks to you, I think I will be able to keep my faith in men."

After the finale of traditional Japanese music, the woodcutter leaves the gate into the sunlight, with the infant in his arms. It is clear, from what we have observed, that the symbolic transition from darkness to light signifies that altruism offers a potential for harmony even in the fragmented world of *Rashomon*. At the same time this transition signifies that man's nature is melioristic as found in the woodcutter's behavior.

However, the last two shots significantly modify this critical deduction. First, Kurosawa presents a long shot from behind the woodcutter as he walks into the sunlight in vivid contrast to the shadow over the gate. Then the camera swiftly moves to a long shot of the woodcutter from the opposite angle. As he walks toward the camera, he stops and bows to the priest, beaming with happiness. However, despite the woodcutter's magnificent display of optimism, we are visually deluded, for now we are given the impression that the woodcutter is walking into the shadow while the whole gate and the clear sky come into frame behind him.

This reversal of the light and darkness, the shadow and sunlight, which has hitherto been neglected by Kurosawa's critics, seems to deny the optimistic tone with which most viewers see the film end. Rather, it stresses the difficulty of maintaining a melioristic stance in the fragmented world. Concerning the ending of *Rashomon*, Kurosawa himself says that he wanted to present gigantic columns of clouds (cumulo nimbus) above the gate, but they never appeared

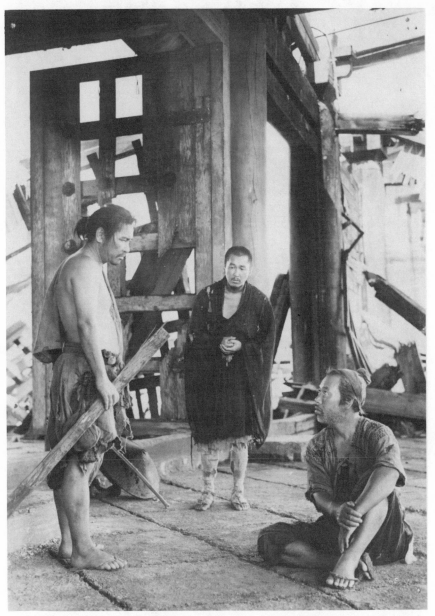

Rashomon (1950). The commoner (Kichijirō Ueda), the priest (Minoru Chiaki), and the woodcutter (Takashi Shimura) at the gate.

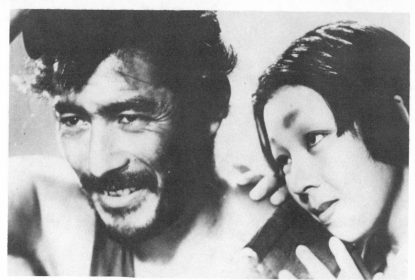

Rashomon (1950). The bandit Tajōmaru (Toshirō Mifune) and Masago (Machiko Kyō).

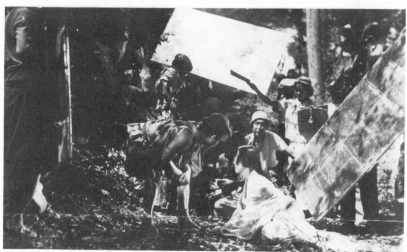

Rashomon (1950). Akira Kurosawa directing Toshirō Mifune and Machiko Kyō.

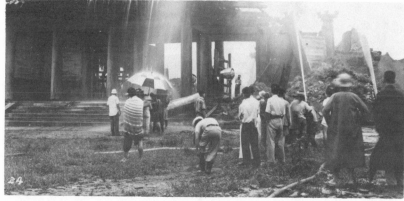

Akira Kurosawa and his staff on the set of the Rashomon Gate.

during the shooting of the final scene.⁹ The image of cumulo nimbus predicting approaching rain, though an external datum, serves as another justification for supporting the relativity of man's nature as the film's final implication.

NOTES

1. Akira Iwasaki points out that in spite of the Western and the Japanese that coexist in Kurosawa, he "belongs to a more recent generation which must look to the West for help in describing Japan." According to Iwasaki, in *Rashomon* and his other movies Kurosawa is concerned with things "unusual, non-routine or abnormal" and tries to convey the inner significance of the story, in strong contrast with such "Japanese artists" as Ozu and Naruse, whose themes are concerned with daily events in the traditional Japanese society. See "Kurosawa and His Work" in *Focus on Rashomon*, ed. Donald Richie (Englewood Cliffs, N.J.: Prentice-Hall, 1972), pp. 21–31.

2. Satō's criticism focuses on the rhythmic movement of the scene in which the bandit assaults the wife, while the husband watches. Satō, enumerating the fourteen different shots that are employed for this scene, describes the significance of the impressionism of the sunlight, which reveals "the naked humanity" of assailant and victim. See *"Rashomon"* in *Focus on Rashomon*, pp. 95–102.

3. For example, Parker Tyler, referring to Kurosawa's dexterous use of the flashback technique, states that the different versions of the story given by the characters point to "the traumatic violence of the basic pattern: that violence which is the heart of the enigma." See *"Rashomon as Modern Art"* in *Focus on Rashomon*, pp. 129–39.

"Rashomon" by Donald Richie is the most comprehensive study of the film from the viewpoint of its philosophical implication, its cinematography, and the development of the filmic action. Richie states that Kurosawa's main concern in this film is with the rendition of the subjective reality and the exploration of the concept that human beings cannot judge "reality much less truth." See *Focus on Rashomon*, pp. 71–94.

4. Tadao Satō makes a significant remark that throughout the history of Japanese cinema, the social milieu of the Heian period, which is the temporal background of *Rashomon*, has never been the cinematic focus of any director. It is Kurosawa who has proved that the social milieu of this period provides aspects significant enough to form what we call "aristocratic" ("ōchō") genre. See *Nihon Eiga Shisoshi* [The History of Intellectual Currents in Japanese Cinema] (Tokyo: Sanichi Shobō, 1970), pp. 312–13.

5. According to *Mappō Shisō* [The Theory of the Last Phase of the Law], which was circulating during the Heian period, 1,550 years after the death of Buddha, Buddhism will enter into a descending cycle. In this last phase of Buddhism, the degeneration characterized by the complete disharmony between Buddhist preaching and its proof takes place. There are multiple theories on the beginning of the last phase of Buddhism, and one theory asserts that it is supposed to begin at the end of the ninth century.

6. Richie, *Focus on Rashomon*, p. 87.

7. Marcia Landy, "Film and Politics: A Review of Selected Films by Akira Kurosawa," p. 11. Paper presented on the panel, "Focus on Kurosawa Films," at the Mid-Atlantic Conference of the Association for Asian Studies (October 1978).

8. Richie, *Focus on Rashomon*, p. 88.

9. Akira Kurosawa, *Akuma no Yō ni Saishin ni: Tenshi no Yō ni Daitan ni* [Be careful as the Devil: Daring as an Angel] (Tokyo: Tōhō, 1975), p. 120.

2

Sand, Man, and Symbols: Teshigahara's
The Woman in the Dunes

Since 1962 Hiroshi Teshigahara has been adapting the novels of
Kōbō Abe for films and like Abe, has pursued existential themes.
The Pitfall [Otoshiana, 1962], an avant-garde film based upon a
television drama script by Abe, was Teshigahara's first feature film.
He went on to screen *The Woman in the Dunes* [Suna no Onna,
1964], *The Face of Another* [Tanin no Kao, 1968], and *The Ruined Map*
[Moetsukita Chizu, 1968], all of which are also faithful renditions of
Abe's novels. Among these films, as Donald Richie and many other
critics have pointed out, *The Woman in the Dunes*, winner of the 1965
Cannes Festival First Prize, is undoubtedly the finest, distin-
guished by its skilled photography and unique symbolism.

The protagonist's entrapment in the sand in this film has been
interpreted in several ways. One of Japan's leading critics, Tadao
Satō, explains the protagonist's dilemma from the perspective of
the assaulter and the assaulted.[1] Donald Richie sums up the film as
an exploration of "the search for identity,"[2] a motif that runs
through Abe's many novels. Both Kyōichirō Nanbu and Tadao
Satō point up some challenging and pivotal questions to which the
director has addressed himself:

> This is truly a strange film. Why on earth does the woman keep
> digging away at the sand in the pit? Why can't the man (Niki) escape
> from it? The more one thinks about it, the more complex the situation
> appears. We do not understand what the characters are doing. But
> perhaps life is just as unfathomable; the basic question is, after all, why
> one lives in the first place. Some viewers will of course draw particular
> allegories from the film. It might suggest to them, for example, that
> once man recognizes life as merely a repetition of meaningless actions,
> like digging at a sand dune, it can sometimes be surprisingly interest-
> ing.

Others may interpret the film as an exposition of the relationship between engineers (the man and the woman) and politicians (the villagers). The sand, in any case, represents a platitudinous existence that overwhelms human beings with stark, awesome pressure. The sense of unexplainable oppression is the sole merit of this film.[3]

The viewer of *The Woman in the Dunes* cannot help but notice the importance of texture; the film is replete with cinematic metamorphoses of sand that create vibrant, sensory impressions. At the beginning, Teshigahara presents a vast stretch of sand, like a rippling ocean. In one scene, a single magnified grain of sand fills the entire screen; in another, sand flows on and on in a white cascade. In order to emphasize the inseparable bond between the two main characters (Niki and the sand woman) and the sand—their environment—Teshigahara films the sand so that it becomes a part of their very corporeal existence. Thus the variegated pattern of the sand is projected on both characters. Its rippled pattern is duplicated in the design of the woman's blouse. Her voluptuous body, especially her hips, move with the undulations of shifting sand. In a close-up of the protagonist's naked back, grains of sand adhere to his skin like innumerable beads of sweat. The woman, naked, is covered with sand, distinctly outlining the curves of her body. Inanimate sand, always moving through these metamorphoses, becomes as animate as the *dramatis personae* and gradually commands closer attention from the viewer.

The first step in an analysis of this difficult film is to examine the presentation of the bond between the sand as environment and the protagonist. This means we must study the nature of the protagonist's response to the flowing sand, the woman, and the villagers of the dune community. From there we may go on to analyze the implications of the sand symbols and the protagonist's actions.

The film begins with images of the countless officially stamped cards and documents an individual must carry on his person. Then a grain of sand magnified many times fills the screen accompanied by the sound of sharp, resonant knocking. The following sequence shows trickling sand, and then a human figure, struggling alone, intruding upon the scene. The figure removes his shoes, shaking out the sand. This man moving slowly along the ridge of the dune is Niki, apparently an insect collector. Reflecting earlier shots of the sea below the dunes, the camera now captures the smooth rippled patterns of the sand. Then, as the clear outlines of Niki's footsteps interrupt the ripples, Teshigahara introduces the man's unavoidable association with the sand.

At an early stage, the director establishes the basic quality of
sand: aside from its endless metamorphosis, that quality is its corrosive power. The protagonist's attention focuses suddenly on a patch
of dried-up grass in the lee of a rotting fence. The grass is withered
from lack of water, and the fence is corroded. Niki continues his
journey across the dunes;[4] as the sun sets, he is but a dot on the vast
expanse. This tiny figure is in trenchant contrast to an earlier shot
of an insect filmed in close-up and blown up many times its actual
size; it is a comment on the insignificance of human life amid the
immensity of predatory sand that absorbs everything which rests
upon it.

The camera again captures the lone figure of Niki trudging along
the dune, foreshadowing the theme of quest in the film to be
clarified a few scenes later. Niki's path passes a boat half buried.
The liquid quality of sand, illustrated earlier in the simile of ripples
of ocean and sand, is proved an optical illusion. The camera reveals
the sand's heavy, absorbent power; nothing can float or sit upon it.
Niki sits in the boat and muses:

> People need so many certificates just to confirm themselves against
> each other: Contract, License and I.D. Card, Usage Permit, Deed,
> Permit. Registration and Permit to Carry. Union Card. Letter of Com-
> mendation. Promissory Note. I.O.U. . . . Temporary Permit. Written
> Consent. Income Certificate and even Pedigree. . . .
> That can't be all.
> Aren't there any more?
> Haven't I forgotten to certify something?
> Where do they end?
> The certificates go on and on. . .[5]

From these images and that of the official stamps introduced at
the beginning of the film, we immediately understand that Niki's
daily life is regulated by thousands of certificates, a motif common
in Abe's novels. Here, in film, the director observes that a socially
fabricated identity governs contemporary man; alienation is inevitable even in the smallest social unit, the family. In a sequence
where his wife appears, Niki, in a voice-over, reveals his domestic
unhappiness: "You criticized me for arguing too much. But this is a
fact!"

Niki's journey along the sand dune and his reflections on his
daily life have already stated the central problem of the film: "How
can contemporary man come to terms with society?" The sand
itself is society, and Niki must confront it, trapped in the dune.

What takes place after Niki's confinement in the sand dwelling is the dilemma of options—escape to his former life or resignation to life in the sand pit—and its resolution. Throughout the remainder of the film, the dliemma is dramatized by Niki's gradual shift away from the first option toward the second. An examination of the dominant images in the sand pit and Niki's relationship to both the sand and the sand woman, as well as to the villagers, provides a key to the thematic development of his dilemma. Before accepting the sand pit as his final choice, the protagonist attempts to escape four times.

In detail, Teshigahara portrays life in the sand pit prior to the first attempt, characterizing the sand as a menace to human existence. As he descends into the sand dwelling, intending to stay only overnight, Niki perceives how decrepit the walls of the house are, and that its beams are misaligned. The sand has besotted and rotted the straw mats *(tatami)*. The woman wears traditional Japanese trousers with a ripple pattern, again reminding us of her closeness to the sand. Otherwise, she has no name and no "socially fabricated" identity.

The subsequent film action and dialogue between the man and the woman reveal in realistic detail how anyone inhabiting the place is utterly unable to escape from the creeping power of the sand. The woman puts up an oil-paper umbrella while Niki eats dinner to keep the sand from falling into his food. When he finishes eating and takes down the umbrella, he is astonished at the volume of sand that pours off it. While they are eating, the woman explains that the sand rots things so quickly that even a new pair of wooden clogs is ruined in a month or so. But Niki protests stubbornly that the notion of damp sand is very strange to him; he has always associated sand with the desert and hence, with dryness.

As the action proceeds, Teshigahara shows the primitive qualities of the sand dwelling. The woman tells Niki that he can have a bath only every three days. A single oil lamp serves as illumination. Upon awakening the following morning, Niki finds the woman asleep completely naked. The camera captures his surprise at the sensuality of the naked woman, who looks like a statue covered with sand. The activities of night and day are reversed in the sand pit; at night the woman is active, digging at the sand while it is damp and manageable.

Niki's first attempt to escape takes place that morning. The camera focuses on the outside of the house, catching the sun and scorched sand. Niki emerges to find that the ladder is gone. The steep, wall-like sand slope is threatening as he stands beneath it. Trying to climb out, he finds himself after several steps sinking into the sand and slowly, helplessly sliding back to his starting point. As he asks the woman for a ladder, part of the sand wall collapses onto and shakes the house. Teshigahara's camera brilliantly catches the waterfall-like flow of sand.

At this stage, the two options that compose the central problem become clear to us: imprisonment in the sand dwelling requires one to constantly fight its encroachment by digging away every night. Escape means leaving the pit and returning to society. At this point, Niki chooses the second alternative. He frequently expresses his yearning to return to his own society by alluding to time, around which society organizes life. After his first night in the sand dwelling, he looks at his wristwatch, which reads 11:16. Protesting the absence of the ladder, he says bluntly to the woman: "I am a person with a job. And therefore I want to use my time with care."

Niki's second attempt to escape from the sand pit is also futile. Panting and perspiring, he starts shoveling a path forward. Directed from the woman's perspective, as she watches him, the camera catches three heads peering over the rim of the pit. These heads, tied with kerchiefs of working men, are filmed as a threat to Niki, their expressions furtive and sneering. As he continues to dig, the sand slides suddenly down in a rushing stream, ultimately striking him down. This sequence evokes the symbolic destructive power of sand, once again being reinforced. The audience now comes to realize that the sand is an index of society, a monolithic dynamic that subjugates its individual components. Society is not inert. Just as sand asserts its tyranny in diverse forms—a cataract, a stream, the sea, a magnified single grain—society overwhelms the individual in many ways. It demands that the individual conform on its terms. As yet, however, Niki's perspective on his predicament is so limited that he cannot grasp the true nature of sand (society). Therefore, he still associates the outside with limitless freedom, and the sand dwelling with imprisonment.

Niki's third attempt to find a way out of the sand pit is also futile. Stuffing a towel into the woman's mouth and tying her hands and legs, he tries to use her as a means of escape. He cries to the villagers above the pit to pull him up: "If you want to save her, pull me up right now."

The camera pans the rim of the pit from the villagers' perspective, over the man and house, objectifying the relationship between victimizer (sand and the villagers above) and victim. The house appears flattened from above; its roof dominates the screen. Niki, looking helplessly up at the rim, is diminutive in the expanse of sand. A sense of claustrophobia comes through the film, conveying the feelings of a victim taunted by society to which he still desperately reaches out, oblivious to its true oppressive nature. The victim's predicament is intensified by falling sand, which prevents him from looking up. In order once more to impress upon the viewer the dehumanizing aspect of society, Teshigahara presents the man completely at the whim of the villagers above, who manipulate the rope he clutches. They pull him up about five feet, then suddenly let go. The man tumbles back into the sand pit. Now from below we hear low chuckles become loud, derisive laughter. The rope, symbolic of the false hope of freedom, reduces the individual to a helpless victim; society refuses him freedom on *his own terms*.

After showing Niki in three unsuccessful attempts to escape from the sand pit, Teshigahara begins to portray the steady erosion of his reason and emotion. Once Niki decides to give up his reliance on time, he finds himself physically attracted to the sand woman. The camera articulates her sensual qualities, focusing on the contours of her body, especially her curving hips. The woman is frequently filmed in the shadow of the house, emphasizing the association of erotic qualities with darkness.

The constant threat of the sand to human existence is visible everywhere in the pit, as Niki gradually admits: "It's useless to fight it! The thing called sand, if it wants to, can swallow up a city or even a country, just like that!" But until he experientially perceives the true nature of the sand, he cannot suppress his yearning for liberation from the sand pit. Trying still again to escape, he rips wood off the wall of the house to make a ladder. The woman tries to stop him and they wrestle. During the struggle her breast is exposed and he accidentally touches it. A fierce sand slide overwhelms them, like pouring rain.

As Niki's reason and emotion are slowly sundered, he responds to impulse, now portrayed in his sexual arousal. The woman removes her clothes and brushes off the sand with a towel. As she kneels down, moving her hand from her neck down, the camera, like Niki's eyes, is fixed on her back. In the following scene, as Niki and the woman make love, her moving body is filmed to highlight its similarity to the undulating flow of sand. Her toes sink into the sand, and Teshigahara's camera details the beads of sweat mixed with sand on Niki's bare shoulders. Grains of sand seem to seep even into human skin. This scene suggests the inescapable threat of

sand; society sifts even into the very core of human existence—the
love between man and woman—thus dooming every individual to
alienation. Neither the sand woman nor Niki can allow the flow of
the sand to overwhelm them. Both must constantly dig at it in
order to survive.

The protagonist's fifth attempt to escape takes place after he has
made a rope. He makes the woman drink some sake, causing her to
fall into a deep sleep. He then climbs onto the roof, from where he
hurls the rope toward the rim of the pit. After a number of unsuccessful attempts, Niki finally throws the rope over a heavy bag at
the rim. The camera panning from above as he throws the rope
catches the desperate enthusiasm of his hope for freedom. In strong
contrast to the sky, filmed white to suggest sought-after freedom,
the sand slope appears in ominous black silhouette—a deadly
menace. Niki pulls at the rope to test it, and discovers that it will
hold his weight. He struggles upward as the sand pours over him
and sweat runs into his eyes.

Having climbed at last out of the pit, Niki thinks he can simply
walk to freedom. On a symbolic plane, his escape can be interpreted as an effort to integrate himself into society on his own
terms, but the following scenes reveal an ironic twist. The real
nature of society is not what he had expected; it affords him no
freedom after all. By investing the sand dune with disorderly and
destructive qualities, Teshigahara again projects the monstrous
hostile power of society. A violent wind blows along the dune.
Before Niki stretches an endless expanse of barren and reddish
sand, quite unlike the soft flowing undulations shown before. The
sand blows constantly into his eyes and frustrates his progress.
Stinging grains of sand cling to every inch of his skin. He sights the
ridge of the dune, which reflects the sun in gold. We might associate this light with the goal of his journey, the promise of an
individual freedom. But the shining light on the ridge suddenly
disappears, to be replaced by a gray mist. To reach his goal may be
impossible after all.

We watch Niki journeying along the sand dune, panting, his feet
dragging. The night comes and in the heavy darkness barking dogs
conjure up horror and confusion. He starts running randomly, and
then realizes that the three flashlights he sees in the distance are his
pursuers. His escape is cut off as he becomes trapped in quicksand.
The more he struggles, the deeper he sinks in. He cries desperately
for help. Several inhabitants of the sand community, cheerful and
joking, drag him out while he writhes in agony and fear. The

indifference and hostility of the villagers as they silently toss him back into the pit reflect the impersonal relationship of individuals to society.

Niki escaped from the sand pit only to be trapped in the even more formidable accumulation of sand outside. So the endless dune at the beginning of the film returns—a colossal stretch of sand that absorbs the protagonist.

In the following scene Teshigahara presents the moths and other insects that Niki collected as an entomologist. The irony lies in the shared fate of the tiny insects pinned down to the board and the entomologist who pinned them there. Both are helpless victims; just as the insects are classed into some genus and species, so is man forced into a socially fabricated identity. Like the insects, the man is pinned down by the forces of society. This scene cuts quickly to outside the house as if not to let us forget Niki's entrapment.

In order to impress upon the audience the impossibility of Niki's attaining limitless freedom in society, Teshigahara now introduces a symbolic flock of crows. Niki digs a hole to trap them.

MAN: It's hope.
WOMAN: Hope?
MAN: It's a trap for crows. I attach bait here . . . As soon as a crow takes it in his mouth, you see, he'll be sucked down helplessly along with the wind.
WOMAN: But crows are smart though . . .
MAN: When they get hungry, they get stupid.
WOMAN: But why did you say it was hope?
MAN: (Continues working). It's hope. I will attach a letter to the leg of a crow I catch. Asking for help . . .
WOMAN: (Laughs a little) Really! It hasn't come. It has been almost three months . . .
MAN: What hasn't . . .?
WOMAN: Help.⁶

We can predict that no crow will be caught and that Niki's goal of liberation from the pit will not be achieved. This bird, which the Japanese associate with death, is far from a symbol of "hope." Escape from imprisonment, which Niki equates with hope and which becomes his soul, is apparently only a false goal.

Even at this stage the protagonist still does not see that the external world, which he believes is the realm of freedom, is actually the realm of bondage. In vain he still pleads with the villager who has thrown down a package:

Wait a minute! Will you let me go out for a short time? . . . Once a day, even for only thirty minutes . . . I want to see the sea! Please . . . I promise . . . I definitely won't do anything like running away! Twenty minutes, or even ten minutes will do . . . I have been obedient for three months already . . . Please! I'll go out of my mind![7]

Until he finally reconciles himself to his predicament as contemporary man, Niki is inevitably in conflict with the external world. This confrontation is expressed in his direct conflict with the villagers who are looking down at him and the woman from the edge of the pit. A torchlight carried by one of the villagers imparts a ghostly nocturnal atmosphere to the scene while at the same time it conveys the claustrophobia of the man below. The villagers tell Niki to make love to the woman while they watch in return for safe passage out of the sand dwelling. Precisely at that moment the internal conflict within Niki—conflict between reason and emotion—comes to a climax. This conflict is objectified by two sets of characters: the sand woman telling him that he cannot possibly commit himself to such shameless conduct, and the villagers, who insist he fulfill their demand:

MAN: What shall we do?
WOMAN: (without looking up) Ridiculous!
MAN: But at least it's an opportunity . . .
WOMAN: Ignore them.[8]

Emotion overwhelms reason, and he sweeps the woman to the ground.

The following sequence illustrates the climax of his confrontation with the external world. The villagers' faces are suddenly transformed into sinister devil masks. Figures of the villagers in white kimonos carry torchlights, and begin to dance to gradually intensifying drumbeats. Only the torches and white kimonos stand out against the black background, and the atmosphere grows orgiastic. This unique expressionistic technique serves to project the protagonist's inner feelings onto the screen. Within his consciousness the external world becomes a distorted and monstrous entity that forces even the commercialization of sex upon the individual. The woman kicks Niki hard in the stomach, and crouching, starts pummeling his head. Her cry, "Fool! Fool! Fool! Fool! Fool!" finally brings him to his senses.

The next scene takes place the following morning. Niki is standing outside the house, with a vacant expression on his face. Above, the crows, so much freer than he, seem to mock him for failing to escape. A gusting wind blowing against the house highlights his gloom. Lifting the lid of the bucket he had set as a crow trap, which he named "Hope," Niki is surprised to find that it is full of water. Suddenly he realizes that capillary action has extracted water from the sand. For him too, a process of distillation takes place. He then understands the metaphysical implications of this phenomenon; that his predicament is that of contemporary man!

Prior to this revelation, Niki experiences a spiritual growth that is thematically of equal importance: the germination of love between him and the sand woman. She has been busily stringing beads so that she can buy a radio. The radio suggests not only the dissolution of the communication barrier between the two but also the inception of communication with the external world. Although Niki still hopes to find a means by which to extricate himself from the sand pit, Teshigahara's images foreshadow the man's ultimate acquiescence to life there. Niki's allusions to time become less frequent, and eventually his watch, the last bond to the society to which he wants to return, stops. For Niki and the woman there is only the present, and her remark, ". . . until tomorrow . . ." is meaningless. Before his last escape attempt Niki burns his insect collection. The equation of the insects with himself, a social insect, is thus nullified. The gesture indicates his chosen course of action: repudiation of his artificial identity.

As these images unfold—the dissolution of time, the denial of a socially fabricated identity, and finally the almost primitive love between the man and the sand woman—the final implication of the sand pit becomes obvious. This is a record of man's centripetal journey to his inner self, the nucleus of basic human emotions. Man consists of an inner self, which is true to his fundamental nature, and an outer self, which wears a social mask. The flaking mirror, filmed close-up, is indeed the analogue for man's confrontation with his inner self. In society, where the mirror functions properly, man sees only the reflection of his social mask. The fight against the corrosive, all-enveloping sand represents contemporary man's continuous striving to preserve his inner nature against a dehumanizing society by refusing to wear the social mask. Abe suggests that love between a man and a woman has the potential to create a better world, in that it mitigates man's alienation.

Even this, however, is obviously too easy a solution. The child the woman conceives, a symbol of a better future, must be aborted because she has an extrauterine pregnancy. Against her will, she is drawn up out of the pit on a rope to be taken to the hospital. Again the menacing power of the sand is evoked as it starts pouring down on the helpless woman. Her plaintive cry, "No . . . No . . . No . . ." gradually fades away.

Next is a close-up of the rope ladder left behind. Alone, Niki is now free to escape. He grasps the ladder lightly and starts climbing up. When he finally comes out into the open air, the mountainous stretch of sand again appears threatening. The sky is desolate and a strong wind whips up the sand. He walks several steps, and then notices that not even the sea is soothing. He suddenly realizes that the external world is not as he had conceived it while desperately struggling to escape from the sand pit.

The following scene, marking the moment of his epiphany, shows Niki returning voluntarily to the confinement of the sand dwelling as he knows now that only there can he remain faithful to his inner self and that only there can true, if somewhat attenuated, freedom be found. This scene opens as Niki slowly begins to climb down the ladder. He opens the lid of the crow trap bucket, "Hope," shoving away the accumulated sand. As he discovers that the bucket is full of water, his face is reflected in it. He puts his hand into it.

The sequence articulates in images Niki's discovery of the plight of the individual in the totality of sand, that is, the colossal totality of society. Abe says in his novel: "The change in the sand corresponded to the change in himself,"[9] and the change in the protagonist is his new perspective on life: his willing acceptance of what he had hitherto misconceived as the limitation of the sand dwelling. Having become aware of the threat of society to his very existence, he sees that life will only be meaningful if he preserves his intrinsic human nature, his inner self. Furthermore, having discovered a source of pure water, the basis for survival, Niki need not regard the villagers as hostile. On another level, the water source serves as an index of the motivating force behind his vision of an ameliorated world: the force of love between man and woman. The woman's miscarriage certainly signifies the difficulty of achieving a better world, but the film seems to say that the contemporary man's constant effort to maintain love is more important than the achievement of the goal itself. In this sense, the film presents a rather orthodox solution for a constructive value system.

The following morning Niki remarks to himself, after inspecting the bucket:

There's no need to run away yet. My return ticket will be good anytime I wish to go back. Also, I'm dying to tell somebody about the reserve equipment. I've got to! If anyone, there's probably no one more interested than the people of the village. If not today, maybe tomorrow. I'll think about escaping after I've told someone about it. Maybe the day after.

The viewer now knows that Niki will never leave the sand dwelling; there is no need for a return ticket. His eagerness to tell the villagers about the water reveals his desire for congenial human relationships, which might add some positive value to a life always aware of alienation. This potential is emphasized by the radio Niki is holding in his hands.

The Woman in the Dunes ends with the "Adjudication of Disappearance," which discloses to the audience the protagonist's name, Junpei Niki, for the first time. The court decision states that Junpei Niki is officially designated a missing person. This impersonal legal document impresses the viewer with the victim-victimizer relationship between a fabricated identity (the individual) and society. Yet, undercutting this matter-of-fact treatment of the callousness of society, the film's end seems to celebrate contemporary man's courage to fight the encroachments of society, however absurd his personal battle may be.

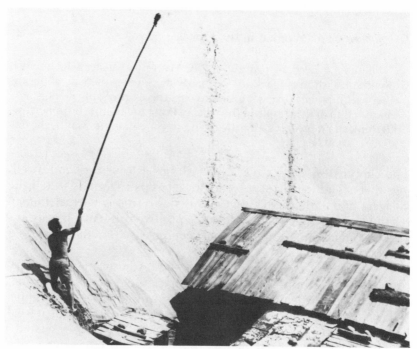

Woman in the Dunes (1964). Niki (Eiji Okada) in the dunes.

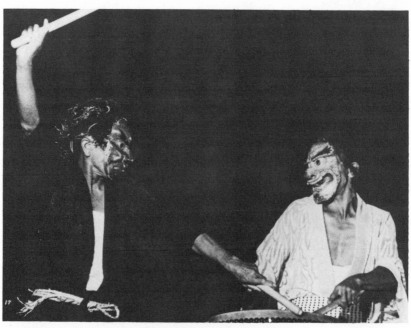

Woman in the Dunes (1964). The masked villagers above the dunes.

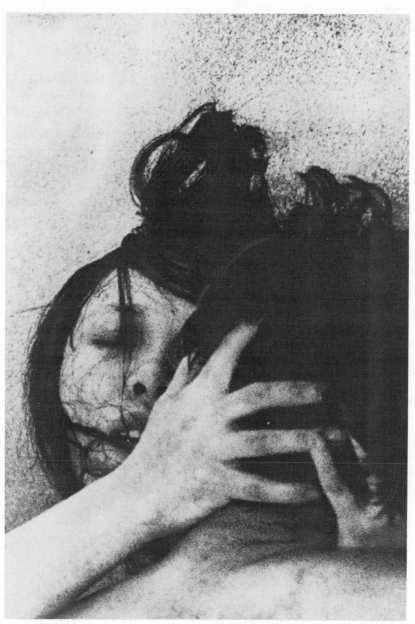

Woman in the Dunes (1964). The woman (Kyōko Kishida) and Niki.

NOTES

1. Satō compares *The Woman in the Dunes* with Yoshishige Yoshida's *Escape from Japan* [Nihon Zasshutsu] and points out that the protagonists in the two films share a certain sense of life's want of fulfillment. See *Gendai Nihon Eiga* [Contemporary Japanese Films] (Tokyo: Hyōronsha, 1976), 1:135–36.

2. Donald Richie, *Japanese Cinema: Film Style and National Character* (Garden City: N.Y.: Doubleday Anchor, 1971), p. 200.

3. Tadao Satō and Kyōichirō Nanbu, *Nihon Eiga Haykusen* [One Hundred Selections of Japanese Cinema] (Tokyo: Akita Shoten, 1973), p. 200.

4. Judith Shatnoff is attentive enough to perceive the lack of horizon in the sand dune, one of its significant features. However, she fails to deduce its implications. See *Film Quarterly* 18 (Winter, 1964–65):44.

5. The text of the film may be found in English in Hiroshi Teshigahara, *Woman in the Dunes* (New York: Phaedra, 1971). The translation of this, and other passages quoted in this chapter are made with reference to the Phaedra version unless otherwise noted, pp. 6–7.

6. Teshigahara, *Woman in the Dunes*, p. 64.

7. Ibid., p. 66.

8. Ibid., p. 71.

9. Kōbō Abe, *The Woman in the Dunes*, trans. Dale Saunders (New York: Vintage, 1964), p. 236.

3

Giri, Ninjō, and Fatalism: Image Pattern and Thematic Conflict in Shinoda's *Double Suicide*

Masahiro Shinoda, a representative of the Japanese *nouvelle vague* movement,[1] has made more than twenty-four films since his directorial debut in 1960.[2] Among them, *Double Suicide* [Shinjū Ten no Amijima, 1969] is considered to be his most experimental film. The film is based upon Monzaemon Chikamatsu's puppet play of the same title.[3] Chikamatsu, who brought the kabuki and bunraku theaters to full maturity during the Genroku era (1688–1703), excelled in domestic tragedy. The focal point of this genre is the clash between *giri* (social obligation) and *ninjō* (personal emotion) within individuals in the feudal society in which Chikamatsu lived. A number of Shinoda's predecessors also made films that were inspired by Chikamatsu's domestic tragedies. Among these were Kenji Mizoguchi's *The Crucified Lovers* [Chikamatsu Monogatari, 1954] and Tadashi Imai's *Night Drum* [Yoru no Tsuzumi, 1958].

However, what distinguishes *Double Suicide* from these two film is Shinoda's synthesis of traditional and modern elements. While faithfully exploring Chikamatsu's theme of the individual torn between *giri* and *ninjō*, Shinoda overtly brings in scenes of sexual encounter. He also incorporates both bunraku and kabuki techniques such as the *kurogo* and the rotating screen and invests them with new functions. These aspects of Shinoda's ingenuity have already been treated by a number of Japanese critics. Yet the unique aspect of *Double Suicide* is Shinoda's use of three images; the lattice windows and checked walls, the water, and the *kurogo*. The way Shinoda presents these images is just as crucial as what they signify. Although, at first glance, Shinoda appears to present the same Buddhist world view revealed in Chikamatsu's original, the subtle interaction of these symbols with the film's thematic development, especially in the final sequence, illustrates the entirely different world view. This is one of the aspects of the film that makes Shinoda's version nakedly modern.

These symbols of *Double Suicide* basically evolve around the tension between *giri* and *ninjō* or bondage and freedom. *Giri*, depicted in the film as it was in Chikamatsu's original, is closely connected with the Confucian virtue of family obligation. In both works, family obligation underlies parent-child, husband-wife, and elder brother-younger brother relationships. Jihei owes loyalty not only to his elder brother but also to his uncle and aunt, who took care of him in place of his deceased parents. Family obligation also binds him to the welfare of his children and Osan, who is one of his cousins as well as his wife. The lattice window (which is also a part of the setting in Chikamatsu's play) and checked walls indicate *giri*. An audience steeped in the Japanese cultural tradition will immediately associate the checked design with the door of a feudal prison. Moreover, Shinoda presents these objects in such a way that they evoke claustrophobic feelings as an externalization of feudal restriction upon individual characters.

Freedom is symbolized by the water image. Again Shinoda's representation of this image is subtle. Water not only recurs in its natural form but also appears in configurations. For example, the rippling water of the river that Jihei sees in the opening sequence dissolves into the wavy smoke from a lantern in a pleasure district. Later, the cloud pattern on the *fusuma* door at a geisha house is superseded by the water on the opposite side, when the door rotates. Significantly, the meaning of the water is twofold. First, the water associated with purification implies freedom through death; the sins of lovers who commit double suicide will be washed away by the compassion of a Buddha, and their love will be requited in Heaven. More importantly, as explained later, this assumption that Shinoda has forced upon us throughout the film is suddenly denied at the very end. Second, this traditional meaning of the water image is combined with the modern Freudian implication. Shinoda equates sexual consummation with death in life and life in death, and reinforces sex as the ultimate form of *ninjō*, liberation from *giri*. Thus, the water in its configurated form adumbrates Jihei's sexual encounter.

A third category of image, the *kurogo*, a fatality index, makes the image pattern of the film more complex. In the traditional puppet theater, three *kurogo* serve as manipulators of each puppet and others serve as stagehands. Although they are always present on the stage, the *kurogo* are clothed and hooded in black so as to be as unobtrusive as possible; they never participate in the play itself, for the puppets and not the puppeteers are the actors in the play. On the other hand, Shinoda makes them just as important as the *dramatis personae* themselves. In certain scenes, the chief *kurogo* becomes a silent sympathetic or detached observer of the characters' plight. In others, both the chief *kurogo* and other *kurogo* are active participants in the action, aiding and abetting the characters as they play through the complicated web of their lives. The *kurogo* also frequently represent an objective view that condemns or condones a breach of rationality in individual characters. The chief *kurogo* also plays the part of a seer, who leads both characters and audience to see the mystery of human relationships. Though their functions shift, one of the prime roles of the *kurogo* is as a fatality or inevitability index, as Shinoda himself comments:

> The *kurogo* lead the lovers, compelled to die, to catastrophe. They represent the eye of our camera and also serve as the agent for the viewer, who wants to penetrate into the mystery of the truth of the lovers' plight. And finally they represent the author, Chikamatsu himself. Their ominously black and silent figures might represent the other side of Chikamatsu, who created the anti-social world tinged with the melodramatic concept of double suicide, and who was a great sentimentalist and hedonist.[4]

The opening sequence illustrates the close interaction between these three symbols and the thematic conflict as well as Shinoda's skillful manipulation of audience perspective. The film opens with the *bunraku* chanter's recitation: "Buddha's mercy, a net from Heaven." The passage sung loudly in tune with the powerful *samisen* (used for the puppet play) not only impresses upon us the image of a compassionate Buddha presiding over the world but also prepares us for our emotional involvement in the feudal world of the lovers. But our initial expectation of a clear-cut traditional telling of the story is immediately shattered in the next scene wherein Shinoda cuts to the hustle and bustle backstage of the puppet theater and shows us how it is used for shooting the film. Shinoda has served notice that we are to take up a properly modern attitude to the drama unfolding in front of our eyes, offstage and on. We are not supposed to drift into an easy identification with the lovers. In fact, by reminding us constantly of a certain "staginess" in the drama *as presented*, Shinoda is guaranteeing our "estrangement" in the Brechtian sense.

Drums beat on the sound track as the film opens in the feudal setting. Shinoda's stylistic use of reverse-angle shots is obvious from the beginning. First, we see an empty arched bridge onto which the protagonist, the paper merchant Jihei, enters, showing his back to the audience. When Jihei reaches the top of the bridge, the camera shifts to capture him from the other side coming down the bridge. Then, as he climbs another flight of the bridge walking away from us, a group of white-clothed pilgrims, the source of drumbeats, comes over the bridge towards the camera. Jihei and the pilgrims pass each other with indifference at the center of the bridge. White kimonos are associated, in Japan, with death, because a dead body is shrouded in a white kimono and placed in a coffin. Together with the sinister drumbeats, the pilgrims' white kimonos already provide a strong death image, presaging the catastrophe that will occur later. As Jihei walks toward the camera, his aloofness and obsession, the motives for which we do not yet know, are expressed by his face taken in a medium shot.

In the subsequent scene we learn the nature of Jihei's obsession: he is contemplating a double suicide. Here again Shinoda's versatile camera captures Jihei's emotional plight. First we see a long shot of Jihei standing on the bridge. Then, the camera slowly pans down straight on a group of *kurogo* standing in a circle beneath the bridge. We hear the sound of the water and see these *kurogo* more clearly; they are surrounding the corpses of two lovers who have committed double suicide. One, who appears to be the chief *kurogo*, looks up; following his line of sight, the camera pans up straight and focuses on Jihei looking down at the water.

Four aspects of this particular scene merit our critical attention. First, thematically it has already established the death image as one of the predominant images in the film, thus foreshadowing the double suicide into which Jihei and Koharu are forced. Second, the water image, which is presented here, initiates a recurrent image pattern. As earlier stated, the water image not only recurs in its initial form but also metamorphoses into many configurations. Moreover, this scene introduces the relationship between the characters and the *kurogo*, of whose existence as a fatality index we become gradually more aware. Although unrelated to the film's image pattern, this particular scene is also important because of Shinoda's camera work. The Brechtian detachment created earlier becomes more complex as the rapidly shifting movement of the camera, which Shinoda employs both vertically and horizontally, warns us against assuming any set view of the character's predicament.

As the subsequent emotional and moral quandary confronted by Jihei reveals, the central problem of the film is the problem of reconciling *giri* (social obligation) and *ninjō* (personal feelings) in order to achieve a whole life. Although the film's action presents *giri* and *ninjō* as mutually incompatible, Jihei's circumstances offer him three options. The first is to give up Koharu and stay with his family, thus following *giri*. The second is to sell out his family and redeem Koharu, thus bowing to *ninjō*. The third option is to redeem Koharu and to stay with his family, adopting a golden mean. Jihei vacillates between the two conflicting virtues until he is finally forced into double suicide by direct confrontation with their incompatibility. There are six stages of Jihei's conflict and each stage is explored by Shinoda's apt adaptation of the three distinctive images.

At the first stage of Jihei's inner combat, Shinoda presents him as a victim of passion *(ninjō)*. When the water into which Jihei gazes while standing on the bridge dissolves into smoke from a lantern in the pleasure quarters, the sense of freedom associated with the transient world of eroticism *(ukiyo)* becomes obvious. Jihei walks along the street from the right of the screen to the left, and we see him passing by the lattice windows of pleasure houses, which dominate the screen. The next moment, through one of the lattice windows, we see Jihei walking from the right to the left against the wood-block printlike wall, which forms the background setting. Both the lattice windows and the wall make us aware of *giri* as the objectification of Jihei's consciousness. However, as the camera then proceeds to an unusually long focus from different angles on Jihei walking through the red-light district, we sense him being guided into labyrinthine depths of passion free from ethical bondage.

Suddenly, the candle in one of the pleasure houses is blotted out by a *kurogo* and a freeze frame follows; the pedestrians come to a halt and dead silence prevails. This frame is a shock and keeps us in suspense about what will follow. Jihei appears as the only moving figure in this static setting; he slowly enters the pleasure house. There follows a close-up of a lit candle, another configuration of the water image indicative of freedom. As the camera moves, we discover that the candle is held by the chief *kurogo*. The *kurogo*, who is gifted with the ability to penetrate the mystery of human affairs, lets us witness along with Jihei sexual passion in which man and woman are entrapped. Now Jihei's psychological transition from *giri* to *ninjō* is complete.

In the subsequent scene we encounter Shinoda's overt yet stylized rendition of eroticism, an element that is absent in the Chikamatsu original. From Jihei's perspective we see a naked couple; a man is kneeling in front of a standing woman, and on his back, which directly faces the camera, is spread a fresh tattoo that adds an intensely carnal quality to the scene. Moreover, the wall behind them is a blowup of a wood-block print of a courtesan, which also enhances the sensual, fleeting mood of the pleasure quarters.

The following scene takes on a new dimension of the cinematic action as Shinoda, shifting from reality, pursues Jihei's recollection of sex with Koharu. Through his memory we discover that Jihei's meager means do not allow him to redeem her. Then, still in his recollection, we are shown how the frustration of these two lovers over their forbidden relationship yields to passion. We see Jihei and Koharu surrounded by a group of *kurogo*, who appear to represent the lovers' reason or social conscience, but as soon as the *kurogo* leave, passion overwhelms them. In spite of their attempt to obliterate the feudal restriction of their life in Jihei and Koharu's sexual encounter, we already sense doom in their affair through the director's subtle presentation of images. First, Shinoda lets us see the couple through the lattice window, which is the analogue for social restriction upon the lovers. Next, he uses an extreme high-angle shot to show them engaging in sex on the floor, which is made of wood-block prints. While highly stylized sensuousness is evoked through the director's naked rendition of their lovemaking and through his use of wood-block prints associated with the fleeting world *(ukiyo)*, the camera's position creates a feeling of claustrophobia, which corresponds to the sense of social bondage *(giri)* felt by the lovers.

The second stage of Jihei's inner conflict is marked by his encounter with Koharu's pretended fickleness, which he believes is real. Here Shinoda's employment of the *kurogo* as an index of fate becomes more frequent, and at the same time the equation of the lattice window and the wall with *giri* becomes more opaque through his modes of representation. When Jihei's elder brother, Magoemon, disguised as a samurai, secretly goes to a pleasure house in order to spy on Koharu, the chief *kurogo*, in turn, spies on

Magoemon as if he were fixing the lovers' fate moment by moment through a complex manipulation of human affairs. The chief *kurogo* serves as a link between Koharu and Jihei, who is not yet aware of Koharu's dissimulation. The *kurogo* literally directs a carpenter to the nearby eating place where Jihei is drinking sake so that Jihei overhears his remark that Koharu will be redeemed by a wealthy merchant named Tahei.

In the subsequent scene, crouching in the shadow near the lattice window of the pleasure house, Jihei witnesses Koharu begging the samurai (Magoemon) to help her out, so that she can break up with Jihei. There ensues a close-up of Jihei's sword thrust through the lattice window. The presentation is extremely stylistic. The narrator's chant describes Jihei's distraction and the *samisen* music correspondingly becomes dissonant as if one of the strings were broken. Inside the house Magoemon holds Jihei's hands extended through the lattice while outside the chief *kurogo*, who now represents moral consciousness acting to curb Jihei's irrational impulse, calms him down. Next, Shinoda cuts to a close-up of Jihei's hands tied to the lattice. The lattice window, going beyond the theatrical function as the main prop in the original play, signifies the protagonist's inability to throw off the social restrictions (*giri*) imposed upon him.

This symbolic implication becomes clearer when the scene shifts from the exterior to the interior of the pleasure house. Precisely at the moment when Jihei learns the identity of the samurai, he is forced into acceptance of social obligation by denying his personal needs. The tragic effect of *giri* upon Jihei and Koharu is mounted through Shinoda's use of the *kurogo* and the setting, aided by his subtle camera movement. First, Jihei and Magoemon sit, facing each other, their sitting profiles perpendicular to the camera and set against a striped wall. The extremely rigid symmetrical composition evokes the sense of feudal duty to which Jihei must conform. Jihei takes out twenty-nine letters of avowal of love from Koharu, which he has kept with him for five years, and tells Magoemon to burn them.

Next, the camera rotates ninety degrees, and we see Koharu in tears lying prostrate between Magoemon and Jihei. All three are now set against the rigidly striped wall. By presenting Koharu cornered by the two men and the wall on three sides, Shinoda makes us aware of the hopelessly irremediable condition in which she finds herself. Being loyal of Jihei's wife but in love with Jihei, she is as torn as he is between *giri* and *ninjō*. The tension of the scene of feudal oppression increases as Shinoda approaches the one-scene, one-shot method, reintroducing the *kurogo* as a participant in the lovers' fate. Magoemon begins to count the letters that Koharu and Jihei have exchanged. Among Jihei's letters, which he has taken away from Koharu, Magoemon finds a woman's letter, which turns out to be the letter of Osan, who had previously begged Koharu to give up her husband and fulfill her obligation as a woman. In spite of Koharu's efforts to take the letter back, Magoemon starts reading it. The formalism that Shinoda employs in the following scene is an extremely strong statement of Koharu's double bind. The reciter, in tune with the percussive sound of the *samisen*, explains the identity of the writer in a powerful voice: "A letter from Osan to Koharu," while the chief *kurogo* comes out, shows the letter to the audience, and then helps Magoemon to read it.

To close the second stage of Jihei's conflict, Shinoda introduces the water image. Jihei moves away from the camera toward a silver screen, whose liquid quality Shinoda makes us see. A group of *kurogo*, acting like the stagehands in the puppet play, turns the screen around as Jihei disappears inside. The screen, rotated in a *kabuki* manner, is decorated on the other side with ominous black clouds, another metamorphosis of the water image; it foreshadows Jihei's destiny to suicide as a gateway to freedom. Our conviction of the *kurogo's* being an agent in Jihei's death also becomes firm.

In the third stage of Jihei's conflict we see him shackled by social conventions. The dramatic action opens with cutting from the exterior to the interior of Jihei's shop. Throughout the subsequent scenes Shinoda is good at making us see what is on the wall, what pattern is on the furniture, and what it means. The interior walls of the shop have vertical stripes whereas the bedding in which Jihei is taking a nap has checkerboard patterns. The small screen, from behind which Osan's head appears, has diagonal stripes. The counter, behind which Jihei sits, figuring on his abacus, looks like the lattice-bars of an ancient prison. Thus, the tight architectonics of the setting can be taken as an extension of the sober, rigid feudal society that structures the characters' everyday world. At the same time those formal aspects of the setting provide an ironic contrast to the turmoil of the domestic scene that takes place against them.

Jihei's aunt (Osan's mother) and elder brother (Magoemon), who have heard the rumor that Koharu will be redeemed by a merchant, arrive at the shop to find out whether that merchant is Jihei. When the visitors, Osan and Jihei, are seated, Shinoda employs the diver-

sity of angles and shots that corresponds to the disharmony among
the party created by the rumor. He then consistently uses a
medium shot of the four as the rumor is denied by both Jihei and
Osan. After Jihei writes a letter vowing that he will work harder
and that he will dissolve his relationship with Koharu, we see the
four congenially aligned in the room. Osan sits next to Jihei while
Magoemon sits next to his aunt. On the surface, this harmonious
alignment taken in a medium shot appears to represent a restoration
of family solidarity as Magoemon and his aunt express their contentment with Jihei's reformation and Osan assures them of his
sincerity. However, when this medium shot, approaching the one-
scene, one-shot method, quickly cuts to a close-up of Osan's disturbed face, our doubts about the security of the family solidarity
thus asserted are confirmed. The underlying sense of dissolution
increases, when Shinoda presents Jihei's full profile at the end of
the narrow corridor. He is captured, sandwiched between the oppressive wall behind him and the equally imposing *shōji* screen in
front. The shot visualizes *giri*, which entraps Jihei in his final destruction. Furthermore, Shinoda presents Jihei's house as a one-
room house, eliminating most of the room partitions (not the ones
facing the corridor) such as the *fusuma* and *shōji*.[5] The main reason
for this device is to effect the spatial flow of the camera since
interroom communication in this film is not as important as in other
films, such as Mizoguchi's. Thus, the sudden alignment of Jihei at
the end of the narrow corridor increases our awareness of the
closed-in atmosphere.

In the following scene, Osan accuses Jihei of still being attached
to Koharu. In response, Jihei tells her that he has been deceived by
Koharu, that he cannot stop crying over his humiliation. Osan,
fearful that Koharu might commit suicide to fulfill her obligation to
Osan, confesses this: Osan has written to Koharu, begging her to
give up Jihei.

After this ironic twist is revealed to us, we enter a fourth stage of
Jihei's conflict. We see him trying to reconcile the two forces that
bind him; by redeeming Koharu he would satisfy his personal
needs *(ninjō)*, whereas by staying married to Osan he would fulfill
his social obligation *(giri)*. Only a rich merchant could afford such
an arrangement, as Tahei has said earlier: "Money can buy everything." A merchant of meager means like Jihei must choose. When
Osan says that she will raise money for Jihei to redeem Koharu, he
embraces her behind the lattice window. The recurrent window
image, which now dominates the entire screen, signifies the power

of society that is unwilling to tolerate any deviation from the norm. Osan takes out the money, which she has kept aside to pay to the wholesaler, and also takes all of her and her children's clothes out of the chest. The chief *kurogo*, the inevitability index, calmly helps her to sort out the kimonos, again giving the impression that the characters' fate is not theirs alone.

The fifth stage of Jihei's conflict is his direct confrontation with his father-in-law, his uncle, which makes him realize the impossibility of reconciling *giri* and *ninjō*. After Osan is taken away from the house by her angry father, the chief *kurogo*, again in sympathy with her plight, sadly watches her leaving the house, standing with the two children she has left behind. Thus, we are initiated into the expression of Jihei's agony fully illustrated by the chief *kurogo*, his slow puppetlike gesture and the freeze frame. All hope of reconciling the two forces shattered, the only path open to Jihei is death. A high-angle, long shot shows Jihei standing forlorn at the corner of the house after everybody else is gone; just as he is visually at the corner, so is he metaphorically cornered by social opposition to his private feelings. He walks to the center of the screen, drops his sword, and cries as loudly as possible. A group of *kurogo* surrounds him, now representing the imperturbable forces of fate. A few of them put their hands on his shoulders and he stops crying. The slow movement of the camera, assisted by a gong and a chime, dramatizes Jihei's helpless challenge to *giri*. We see a close-up of the lattice window, an index of *giri*, which closes upon him. Jihei tries to push it down. Behind it he moves like a caged animal. He knocks the small screen and then upsets the lantern. The lattice window filmed slightly askew and the scattered props indicate Jihei's loss of sense, resulting from his frustration. With this introduction of the skewed lattice window, the sense of imprisonment Jihei feels is now complete to us. When he comes closer to the camera, he throws a stack of papers away. Jihei moves like the puppet, whose movement is manipulated for the slow, stylized demonstration of the character's emotion. Capturing the striking contrast of the white paper thrown into the air against a solid gray background, a freeze frame crystallizes Jihei's emotional tension.

After one group of *kurogo* removes the damaged props, another group awaits him. They surround him and, to the accompaniment of the gong, push him through the rotating *fusuma* door (room partition), as if they were manipulators of his fate. The plain silver surface on one side of the door is now replaced by the water patterns on the other side as Jihei disappears. The water image, recalling the opening river scene wherein Jihei was gazing at the two corpses, presages the final outcome of Jihei's action, suicide with Koharu, through which he hopes to achieve their happy reunion after death.

Now that Jihei's conflict has reached its culmination, we are initiated into what we call *michiyuki*, the lovers' journey to death. Both the *michiyuki* sequence and the subsequent scene of double suicide need a detailed analysis for two reasons: first, Shinoda's representation of *kurogo* reaches its stylistic maturity; second, the prolonged conflict between *giri* and *ninjō* is finally brought to resolution in a manner different from Chikamatsu's. In this sequence, the *kurogo's* role grows more prominent, as though it were his responsibility to effect the fate of Jihei and Koharu. After a complete blackout accompanied by a sinister gong, we see the chief *kurogo* on a bridge. He suddenly runs off to hide and secretly watches Koharu sneaking out from a pleasure house to join Jihei. He also watches Magoemon and Jihei's children coming to the pleasure house to inquire about Jihei. As they walk away, unable to ascertain Jihei's whereabouts, the chief *kurogo*, the omnipotent seer of the entire situation, follows them. As if to reassure himself that the children will not be around to interfere in the climax, the *kurogo* stops in the middle of the street and watches them until they disappear into the distance.

Silently followed by the chief *kurogo*, again an inevitability symbol, Jihei and Koharu arrive at the graveyard. While they make love surrounded by tombstones, death, which began the film, meets love, which has been the film's substance. The scene of death in love, or love in death, makes explicit in Shinoda's film a sensuousness that is only implied in Chikamatsu's original. When they embrace in sexual ecstasy silently presided over by the chief *kurogo*, the *samisen* music that has been frantically jumping between high and low tones for some time becomes consonant, expressing their physical union. When Jihei and Koharu awake among the tombstones, the *kurogo's* function radically changes. They now become more active participants in the lovers' fate, assisting in the final act of double suicide. The chief *kurogo*, close by the lovers, watches them cut their hair in the traditional act of separation from society.[6] Then, the scene quickly cuts to a group of *kurogo* surreptitiously following the lovers. When Shinoda cuts back to the lovers' site, it is the chief *kurogo* who now leads them to their destination. The distance between the two parties lessens. The chief *kurogo* beckons to the lovers from the bridge, and they approach him slowly.

Shinoda uses an extreme long shot of the two parties for this bridge scene, placing the camera at an extremely low angle. The fusion of the lovers' tiny figures with their desolate surroundings enhances a sense of their discord with the environment: their alienation.

After Jihei stabs Koharu, the last sequence of the film brings us to Jihei's suicide. In this sequence we witness the director's spatial concern and his more active employment of the *kurogo* as a fatality symbol. The wind comes up and a mist drifts in, providing an atmosphere that externalizes Jihei's feelings. We watch him climbing a hill. The camera then cuts to the top where the black figures of two *korogo* and the scaffold stand against the white sky. The discordant music, composed by Tōru Takemitsu and played by the drum and the *shichiriki*, augments the tension of the scene. A number of *kurogo* put the final touches on the scaffold as Jihei approaches it reluctantly. Subsequently, Jihei's legs hang in the air against the chief *kurogo*. There follows a crosscut of a crowd anxiously running toward the camera. Accompanied by the discordant music that has persisted on the sound track, the *kurogo* put away the ladder and indifferently leave the screen, as if they had completed the final state of their participation in the lovers' fate.

Now in silence, the camera pans up to capture the entire desolate scene of Jihei's suicide; the wind is still blowing, the scaffold, the chief *kurogo*, a barren tree, and Jihei's body hanging in the air are silhouetted against the white sky. Throughout this sequence, the white sky predominates over the black earth, symbolizing the liberation that the lovers hope to attain in heaven. Viewing this composition, we are reminded of the narrator's introductory chant, "Buddha's mercy, a net from Heaven," and we become convinced of the compassion which will allow their soul's repose in Heaven.

The film begins and ends in the same place, emphasizing the water image, an index of the atonement of the lovers' sin. At the beginning of the film Shinoda's camera panned down on a group of *kurogo* beneath the bridge. This time, the chief *kurogo* stands on the bridge; his location once again impresses upon us his function as arbiter of their fate. The camera then captures the corpses of Jihei and Kohar lying in the shallow part of the river. Their bodies are shot from diverse angles. These final shots express the prime irony of the film, which Shinoda has deliberately postponed to the last moment. According to the traditional Buddhist concept, the corpse should be placed with its head toward the west (the way Buddha died) in order to guarantee a happy journey to Buddha's paradise. At the beginning of the film, the lovers' bodies that Jihei saw from the bridge were aligned in this manner. However, in this final take, Jihei and Koharu are aligned in the opposite direction, his head facing her toes. Here, at the last, the traditional expectation of reunion for the lovers in Heaven is contradicted. Suddenly, Shinoda is suggesting that double suicide is too easy a solution to the lovers' moral dilemma.

To understand the effect of this final take on the audience expecting traditional patterns to prevail, we must relate the scene to an earlier sequence in which, typically for the beginning of *michiyuki*, we saw Jihei and Koharu enter an open square with a lantern burning in the middle of it. They lament their fate as the camera stands at a distance, as if to enforce our detachment, our intellectual concentration on the meaning of the events. This one-scene, one-shot approach is counterpointed with a sweeping motion, so important in earlier scenes. Significantly, when the long take yields to close-ups of the lovers' faces, we feel suddenly invited to empathize. Koharu exclaims: "I don't want to die. All I want is to be with you!" The camera moves from her agonized expression in close-up to Jihei (also in close-up), whose agony is intensified by his crying out: "Obligation! Obligation binds us all."

The lovers clearly juxtapose the "demands" of *ninjō* (Koharu) and *giri* (Jihei). Shinoda cannot reconcile the two. Here he conveys the inescapability of *giri* to the audience, speaking through the lovers. From this scene with the lovers we must move to his final denial of the feudalist Chikamatsu's affirmation of heavenly compassion. Shinoda, the modernist, stresses the impossibility of escaping *giri*, both now and after death. It is in this final scene that Shinoda also reveals his view of society as a victimizer responsible for man's fate.

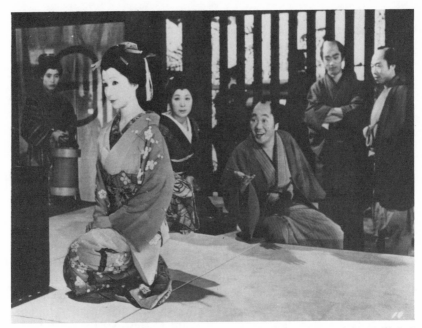

Double Suicide (1969). Koharu (Shima Iwashita) and the merchant Tahei (Hōsei Komatsu) at a teahouse.

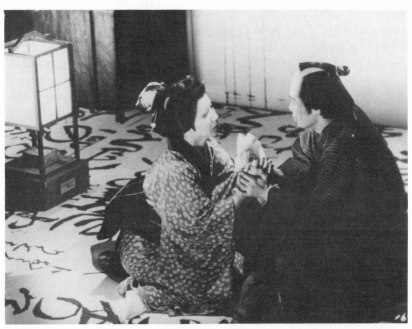

Double Suicide (1969). Jihei (Kichiemon Nakamura) and Osan (Shima Iwashita).

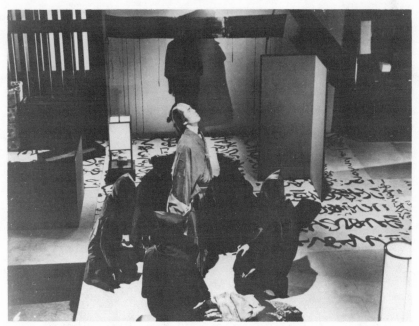

Double Suicide (1969). Jihei (Kichiemon Nakamura) surrounded by the *kurogo*.

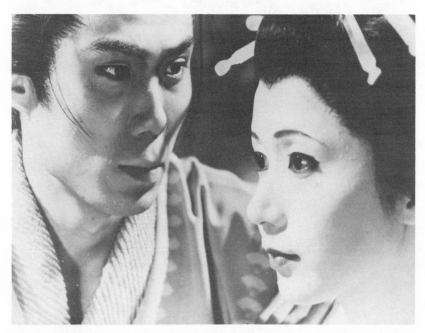

Double Suicide (1969), Jihei (Kichiemon Nakamura) and Koharu (Shima Iwashita) during their journey to death.

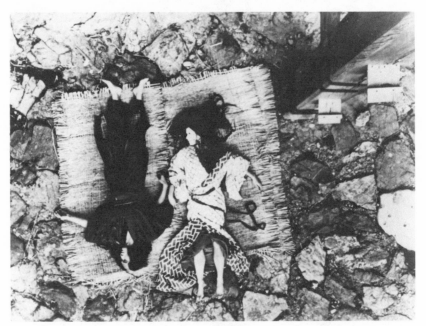

Double Suicide (1969). Jihei and Koharu in the final coda.

NOTES

1. As in France, the Japanese *nouvelle vague* movement was hardly a coherent cinematic movement. The term was loosely associated with a group of directors in the Shōchiku Film Company, who made their debut films in 1960. The major figures in this movement were Nagisa Oshima, Yoshishige Yoshida, Tsutomu Tamura, and Masahiro Shinoda.

2. Apart from *Double Suicide*, Shinoda's representative works are *Pale Flower* [Kawaita Hana, 1964], *Assassination* [Ansatsu, 1964], *Silence* [Chinmoku, 1971], based upon Shūsaku Endō's novel of the same title, a Japanese epic film, *Himiko* (1974), and the most recent work, *Orin Banished* [Hanare Goze Orin, 1978]. Though Shinoda's films encompass the broad historical dimension ranging from the fourth century to the contemporary period, most of his films have one theme in common: the conflict between the individual and the environment that is explored as basically a victim-victimizer relationship. This conflict is quite often presented through his treatment of violence.

3. The English translation of this play is compiled in *Four Major Plays of Chikamatsu*, trans. Donald Keene (New York: Columbia University Press, 1964).

4. Quoted by Tadao Satō in *The History of the Intellectual Currents in Japanese Cinema* [Nihon Eiga Shisōshi] (Tokyo: Sanichi Shobō, 1970), pp. 373–74.

5. For a discussion of the role that the Japanese traditional architecture plays in Japanese cinema, see Noël Burch "On Architecture" in *To the Distant Observer Form and Meaning in the Japanese Cinema* (Berkeley: University of California Press, 1979), pp. 198–201.

6. Traditionally the Japanese cut their hair as part of initiation into nunhood or priesthood, marking their abandonment of the lay world.

Part 2
CHARACTER TYPES

4
Images of Son and Superhero in Kurosawa's *Red Beard*

Red Beard [Akahige, 1965], which is often cited as the most human-istic of Kurosawa's films, has not enjoyed the critical attention that has been given to Kurosawa's earlier major works, *Rashomon* (1950) and *Seven Samurai* [Shichinin no Samurai, 1954]. Donald Richie's study is the only comprehensive work about this film to date. In his study Richie discusses various aspects of the film including the story, the process of production, characterization, and Kurosawa's treatment of such important filmic constituents as symbols, musical motif, and flashback.[1] In *Kurosawa Akira no Sekai* [The World of Akira Kurosawa], Tadao Satō makes a brief yet insightful compari-son of the medical doctor in *Red Beard* with one in *Drunken Angel* [Yoidore Tenshi, 1947]. This suggests further comparisons, which may improve our understanding of character type as a crucial con-stituent of the film.[2]

Akira Kurosawa makes the following comments on film:

> In this movie I only wanted to express the anger manifested in *Red Beard*'s (Dr. Kyojō Niide's) cry, "Did anybody enforce the order that we must not leave human beings ignorant and poor?" And I thought that I had been able to express this anger straightforwardly. I con-sidered this work as the final completion of my works, and I often asked myself what I should direct after this film.[3]

The entire corpus of Kurosawa's filmic works explores his moral and social concerns. His films begin with an acute awareness of a fragmented world, of which the half-ruined gate in *Rashomon* and a dog with a human hand in its mouth in *Yojimbo* are two good examples. Yet man's choices of action in so morally and politically bleak a world are central to his films. As Donald Richie points out,

71

Kurosawa's films present compassion or altruism as offering at least some potential for the betterment of society.

Red Beard begins in true Kurosawa fashion. It is set in a world seemingly governed by forces beyond man's control: the economic destitution of the late Tokugawa period. The story concerns the various stages that a young intern, Noboru Yasumoto, must pass through before he is finally awakened to the greatness of humanism embodied by his chief, Red Beard. The fragmented nature of the world is unfolded gradually rather than presented all at once as in some of Kurosawa's other films. As Yasumoto's perceptions of his surroundings change and enlarge, the seamy aspects of society become more real and immediate.

At the beginning of the film, Kurosawa presents the patients' ward in Red Beard's clinic as a microcosm of the lowest social strata. Yasumoto, returning from Kyūshū after three years' study of Dutch medicine, hopes to be assigned to the Shogun's medical staff. Instead, he finds himself assigned to the public clinic run by Red Beard on a tight budget in shocking circumstances. He is appalled by the poverty-stricken patients who are packed into the dingy quarters of the clinic. We in the audience, who have a much wider perspective than the young intern, already realize that this ward is symbolic of the sickness of society, the worst symptom of which is poverty. With this premise, Kurosawa already posits the central problem of the film, "How can one act in the face of a hostile social environment?"

To explore this central problem, Kurosawa delineates a struggle between two clear-cut value systems: the humanistic confrontation with social evil, a dedication to the public good; and a selfish turning away from social evils, which Kurosawa presents as a bondage to personal aims and understandings.

Kurosawa employs two character types to represent these opposing value systems. Red Beard is the superhero, a man who transcends the prevailing sociopolitical system; a man capable of humanitarian action. He is not only a medical doctor, trying to comfort or cure the poor invalid, but also a psychologist, with some understanding of the emotional sufferings of the poor. Kurosawa invests him with positive human traits: flexibility, fortitude, sense of justice, insight, wisdom, and both physical and spiritual strength. To his young intern, Red Beard (Dr. Niide) is an ideal, and more; he is a father figure. Since curing sick patients serves as an apt metaphor for curing a sick society in this film, Red Beard can be the representative of anyone who is concerned about humanity.

As Red Beard's antithesis, Kurosawa creates the son image in Yasumoto. This young rebel, who at first challenges Red Beard's authority, embodies inflexibility, impatience, self-conceit, and immaturity. Significantly, this dichotomy of character types gradually dissolves as the *son*, in his gradual awakening to the *father's* intrinsic qualities, begins to wish to emulate the father image.

Kurosawa often talks about the rhythmic continuity of his scenario, and as the basis for continuity he alludes either to the *Jo-ha-kyū* pattern of a *Noh* play (Introduction, Development, and Recapitulation at the ratio of 1:3:1) or the symphonic structure.[4] The *Jo-ha-kyū* pattern seems to be more appropriate in this film because it can easily be divided into three parts. The narrative progression of the film is just as straightforward as Kurosawa's character types. The introductory part involves Yasumoto's arrival at Red Beard's clinic and his disgust with his situation and his superior. The second part, the focal point of the film's action, with the turning point at Red Beard's opportune rescue of Yasumoto's life, covers the young man's conversion. It is symbolized by Yasumoto's decision finally to put on the clinic uniform, which he has repeatedly refused to wear. It is in this part of the film that Yasumoto comes to appreciate Red Beard's personality and also to understand the evils of social inequity. The final part of the film, the recapitulatory part and the shortest of the three parts, consists of Yasumoto's affirmation of the importance of humanism. His spiritual learning process has been completed; not only does he demonstrate flexibility in forgiving his ex-fiancée for betraying him but he also shows his dedication by giving up his aspiration to the Shogunate medical staff. In the fusion of the father and son images, this part of the film affirms the potential of humanitarianism for bettering the world.

The first part opens with a shot of the roof tiles of the house in the vicinity of the Koishikawa Public Clinic run by Red Beard. It is raining. A street vendor's voice is intermittently broken by the sound of the wind. Thus, initially establishing gloom as the predominant mood of the film, Kurosawa introduces Yasumoto, an inexperienced, self-centered youth. We see him walking toward the gate of the clinic away from the camera; he stops when he is greeted by Tsugawa, a member of the medical staff. Throughout the film Kurosawa presents this gate as a pivotal point expressive of the various stages of Yasumoto's learning process. At this initial stage, the gate to Yasumoto is just a shabby gate of a public clinic, a place he considers beneath his dignity.

Through Tsugawa, Yasumoto comes to form a false preconception of Red Beard. From this first misconception, Yasumoto begins to mold a negative image of Red Beard as he becomes more acquainted with him. At the gate of the clinic Tsugawa tells Yasumoto that he has been waiting for him so that he can be released from his job. Yasumoto, in dismay, replies that he has simply been advised to go to the clinic to see it. He also proudly says that he has spent three years in Nagasaki studying medicine.

From what little of Yasumoto has been shown us by Kurosawa, we have already learned a lot about him. Yasumoto is somewhat exotically attired as if he were showing off an elite status gained from studying in Nagasaki. His manner, arrogant and conceited, clearly corresponds to his appearance. As the cinematic action progresses, he becomes more and more self-centered. During his stay in Nagasaki in Kyūshū, his teacher, Amano, promised him a position on the Shogunate medical staff. Thus, thinking that he is simply visiting the clinic, Yasumoto exhibits a crude curiosity at the shabby place as if he did not belong there at all. Tsugawa explains to Yasumoto that the medical doctors there are underpaid and constantly put to hard labor by their chief, Red Beard. The camera follows Tsugawa and Yasumoto as they go through the corridor of the outpatient clinic. Yasumoto, with a frown, says blatantly, "What is this smell?" Tsugawa answers: "It is the smell of poverty. . . . This place is frequented by outpatients. Every afternoon, they can receive free medical treatment. . . . These people look as if they would be better off dying than living. . . ." Then, the camera shifts to a crowd of the young, the old, the male and the female—all poorly dressed and crowding into the room. Both visually and verbally, Kurosawa has already presented poverty as the great social evil. He has also made it known to us that Yasumoto must learn to see it as an aspect of social injustice if he is to grow spiritually.

Tsugawa and Yasumoto continue down the long corridor of the ward. In this introductory part, Kurosawa frequently presents Yasumoto walking down the long, dimly lit corridor to foreshadow the long learning process that he will undergo before he finds both his guide and his goal in Red Beard. At this learning stage, Yasumoto responds to poverty as a complete outsider; his response simply remains on a visual level. Thus, he says coldly "Don't you have *tatami* mats around here?" Tsugawa replies that no room in the clinic has *tatami* mats. One of the patients in the ward, pulling his white kimono sleeve, complains that he, much less a female patient, cannot die in such a shabby uniform.

Later, Yasumoto learns that the missing *tatami* and patients' uniforms are part of Red Beard's reforms. Yasumoto believes Tsugawa when he says: "Red Beard is a dictator here. He is very enthusiastic about medical treatment and is indeed an excellent doctor. He enjoys great trust among the feudal lords and rich merchants. However, he is so obstinate, despotic, and extreme. Lately, he has also been acting stuck up." Unable to judge the legitimacy of his informant's description, Yasumoto comes to see his new boss as the very epitome of inflexibility and despotism. But he is doing Red Beard an injustice, as Sakichi, one of the dying patients explains; a *tatami* room is hygienically unsound as it accumulates moisture and dust. Simple white clothes easily show stains so that it is easy to tell when they are clean and hence to keep them more sanitary than colored clothes.

After their tour of the kitchen and staff members' room, Yasumoto has his first meeting with Red Beard. Tsugawa informs Red Beard that he has brought Yasumoto in. We do not see Red Beard but hear his *commanding* voice ordering them to enter. This simple mode of representation signifies that Yasumoto's first impression of Red Beard is formed without his seeing the man. When Tsugawa opens the door, Kurosawa cuts to both Yasumoto and Tsugawa looking at a middle-aged man in a hospital uniform sitting at a desk. All three of them are shown with their backs to the camera. This take magnificently portrays Yasumoto's complete discord with this strange environment, emphasizing the very cold light reflected upon the old *shōji* door and the furniture, and Red Beard's showing his back to the newcomer. Yasumoto's preconceptions about Red Beard are reinforced during this short meeting. Red Beard gruffly introduces himself: "I'm Red Beard." He stares at Yasumoto very intensely, and as if commanding him, he tells Yasumoto that he will start work as an intern at the clinic immediately. Ignoring Yasumoto's objections, Red Beard orders him to hand in all the notes he took during his study at Nagasaki. To the flabbergasted Yasumoto, Red Beard simply says that there is nothing more to discuss. Red Beard then goes back to his desk, showing complete indifference to the two visitors.

As Yasumoto reveals later in a speech to Mori, another doctor at the clinic, his values are entirely conventional; he is a social climber. Thus, Yasumoto arrogantly shows disgust with his assignment to the dingy clinic. Mori quietly tells Yasumoto that the town magistrate, who supervises the clinic, has officially appointed him to the staff at Red Beard's request. At this stage Yasumoto's conceit is so strong that he cannot believe that Red Beard wants his

notes from Nagasaki for the public good. Instead, he thinks that his
boss wants to use them for his own advantage. Furthermore, influenced by his negative impression of Red Beard, Yasumoto refuses to believe that Red Beard treats even those he likes with
something like indifference, even when Mori tells him so.
Yasumoto's fleeting view of Red Beard has been less "telling" than
ours. Kurosawa shows us clearly a keen insight into other people in
Red Beard's glittering eyes but also a humanistic concern for others
beneath his superficially rude manners.

The rest of the cinematic action in this introductory part portrays the impetuous son's open challenge to the tolerant father.
Thus, Yasumoto first must repudiate Red Beard's values to assert
his own until he is brought to see the light. Yasumoto's challenge
manifests itself in his violation of a number of Red Beard's hospital
rules. First, he enters the off-limit area. Kurosawa employs a quick
follow shot as Yasumoto passes through the corridor, then through
the herb nursery on his way to the forbidden building. This follow
shot again emphasizes Yasumoto's long learning process.

In the later scene wherein Red Beard, Mori, and Tsugawa are
seated at the dinner table, Yasumoto refuses to eat. Red Beard does
not scold him at all. Yasumoto's challenge to Red Beard becomes
more violent when he refuses to yield up his notes from Nagasaki.
Yasumoto claims that while he learned advanced Dutch medicine
he contrived his own methods of diagnosis and medical treatment,
and that what he acquired is all his, not anybody else's. Red Beard
loudly responds that medicine belongs to the pubic, not to any
specific person. As early as this stage, we already witness the confrontation of two value systems represented by Red Beard and
Yasumoto, respectively: dedication to medicine versus the exploitation of medicine. Yasumoto, wrapped up in his own world, continues to show his defiance. Against clinic regulations, he orders
the kitchen maid to go and buy sake for him.

Thus, Yasumoto's challenge to Red Beard is not only an independent youth's defiance of authority but also a raving against the
world, which he thinks is not giving him his due. He has assumed
that social advancement would come easily to him for his learning
but not for his professional experience.

Yasumoto's lack of insight into human motives is also manifested
in his inflexibility. He flatly refuses to see Masae, the younger sister
of Chigusa, his ex-fiancée, who betrayed him and married somebody else while he was in Nagasaki. Moreover, he simply idles his
time away in the clinic, disregarding Mori's advice that his childish

attitude is not worthy of sympathy. Significantly, in the final analysis, Tsugawa, who is anxious to leave the clinic for better employment, is what Yasumoto would have become had he not undergone his gradual learning process. Concomitantly, Mori, who is devoted to Red Beard, setting him up as a model, is what Yasumoto might have become had he had a poorer education and a more submissive attitude.

Yasumoto's confrontation with his crushed ego and his subsequent witness to Red Beard's sincere concern for him mark the culmination of the cinematic action of the introductory part. Proud of his acquisition of new medical knowledge in Nagasaki, Yasumoto thinks that he is capable of treating the deranged girl when she escapes from her confinement into his room. Taking at face value her confession that she is not a mad person and that she had to kill her servant for a legitimate reason, Yasumoto encourages her to confess everything to him. While the two sit still, the camera, which has been active so far, becomes almost stationary, externalizing Yasumoto's first professional enthusiasm with the patient, whom he thinks he can cure. This stationary camera position, which has created tension, is ironic; the wind on the sound track during the girl's confession creates a sinister atmosphere, foreshadowing Yasumoto's approaching danger of entrapment in her snare. While the camera is still immobile, Yasumoto approaches the girl closely to show his eagerness. Telling him that she was a helpless victim of rape, she circles around him and then leans against him. Next, the vertical alignment of the two, which the slightly high-angled camera has hitherto emphasized, changes suddenly into a horizontal alignment as she lies down on him and tries to stab him with her sharp hair ornament. This abrupt compositional change, enhanced by a sudden change in the girl's voice, indicates the collapse of Yasumoto's overconfidence in his medical knowledge. It is Red Beard who comes to his rescue just in time.

The following shot presents Yasumoto lying in bed with a white bandage around his neck, which was slightly cut by the girl. The camera cuts to Red Beard's silhouette moving back and forth along the wall. The moving silhouette, more effectively than Red Beard's face in a close-up, conveys his deep concern for Yasumoto, which the youth has not yet come to appreciate. Red Beard now enters Yasumoto's room. Witnessing Yasumoto's embarrassment, Red Beard quickly consoles him, saying that all men have a weakness for a pretty woman. Upon hearing this, Yasumoto cannot stop his tears. Red Beard tries to take a tissue out of his kimono to give to

Yasumoto so that he can wipe his tears, but on second thought he blows his nose with it. A close-up of Red Beard blowing his nose— an amusing gesture to hide his sentimental orientation—indicates his good nature, which is not so frequently shown outwardly or dramatically throughout the film. This episode marks the beginning of the change in Yasumoto's impression of Red Beard.

The second part of the film, the expository part, unfolds Yasumoto's technical and spiritual development, through which he becomes awakened to his moral and professional responsibilities. The first stage of Yasumoto's learning process is his attendance at an operation, wherein he finds his hitherto inflated ego again fatally crushed. When Red Beard asks him to diagnose the patient's illness, he concludes that it is a case of stomach cancer. Red Beard disagrees, telling him that Yasumoto's own notes from Nagasaki show that it is liver cancer. Asked by Yasumoto if there is any cure for this illness, Red Beard answers that there is no way of curing any type of disease. Here Red Beard acts as a mouthpiece for one of Kurosawa's strongest convictions: that poverty and ignorance are the real sources of disease. Red Beard says: "All we can do to compensate for the present poor stage of our medical technology is to fight against poverty and ignorance . . . Everybody says that poverty and ignorance are simply social issues. . . . But have politicians done anything to cure poverty and ignorance? Is there any law that says we must not abandon human beings to poverty and ignorance?"

We have now fully acknowledged that Red Beard is gifted with both medical acumen and empathy for his patients, and that he channels these assets into his actions on behalf of social justice. In the process of becoming, Yasumoto must pass through a series of encounters with clinic patients, who epitomize the sufferings inherent in society. To emphasize Yasumoto's growing sensitivity to his patients, Kurosawa pervasively uses techniques that are easily accessible to the general audience: point-of-view shots, loud music, and flashback. For example, in one scene, three children are brought to the clinic by their mother and are served rice balls in the kitchen. But they are ashamed to show their hunger in the maid's presence, as if this were their childlike defiance of their poverty. As soon as she leaves, they pounce on the food. At this moment Yasumoto passes by the kitchen. They suddenly put the rice balls back on the plate. A medium shot of the children, taken along Yasumoto's line of sight, articulates his impression of these poor children; they gaze at him scared and timid, and huddle together as if fraternity were their sole means of protection. This marks the beginning of his realization of how poverty can deform a child's personality as surely as a disease can deform its body.

Another example is found in the scene of Okuni's confession of her father's (Rokusuke's) gloomy past, through which Yasumoto is awakened to a degree of suffering and misery that his own class is unlikely ever to experience. When Okuni asks Red Beard whether her father died peacefully, Red Beard tells her that her father died a peaceful death. To highlight Yasumoto's perception of Red Beard's insight into his patients, Kurosawa presents (in the intern's recollection) a very quick flashback of Rokusuke's profile on his deathbed while loud music is heard on the sound track. Rokusuke's face, which looked ugly and appalling earlier, no longer looks so to Yasumoto. He realizes that the old man's face expresses the dignity of a man who has silently ended his misery. While the music roars, we recall Mori's earlier remark about his boss: "Dr. Niide can diagnose the patient's body and his mind simultaneously. . . . For example, in Rokusuke's dead silence, he detected terrible unhappiness. . . . That's why he said that his death was solemn."

Yasumoto passes through another stage in his learning process when he witnesses the death of Sahachi, who has always been good to the other patients. Kurosawa again resorts to a series of flashbacks to mark Yasumoto's involvement in the patient's suffering. In the flashback, Sahachi is presented as a good, healy youth, who married Onaka from a poor farmer family. During their happy marriage, a great earthquake devastated Edo, and Onaka suddenly disappeared. A few years later, Sahachi encountered her with somebody else's baby in her arms and learned the truth of her dissimulation; she was afraid of enjoying a happy marriage and thought that a girl like her from a poor family did not deserve to be happy. She saw the devastation of the earthquake—shaking windows, smoke, fissures, and fires—captured by low-key photography in the flashback—as on omen. Sahachi's healthy smiling face at the height of his happiness in the flashback contrasts with his sorrowful, skinny, aged face, and this contrast clearly demonstrates the effects of socioeconomic forces crudely operating in individual lives. Furthermore, the snow-covered farmyard where Sahachi courted Onaka is in stark contrast to the dingy room in the ramshackle house where he is now dying. Again this articulates the innocence of love betrayed by economic determinism.

As Sahachi dies, Yasumoto learns about compassion among the poor for the first time. Deeply concerned about Sahachi's condition, the inhabitants of the slum gather at this house where he was carried from the clinic according to his wish. The pouring rain outside and the torn *shōji* door in the background add a desolate texture to the scene corresponding to their gloom, and the onlookers show genuine sorrow over Sahachi's approaching death. In one scene, the *shōji* is slightly askew, as the house was tilted by a landslide that took place shortly after Sahachi's return. This shot, however, achieves Kurosawa's desired effect in conveying a sense of social inequity victimizing the poor as a feature of Yasumoto's awareness.

The point at which Yasumoto begins to grow is symbolically marked by his decision to wear the clinic uniform. The uniform is the emblem of public service, as evidenced by Sahachi's remarks that when the poor, who cannot afford a doctor, see a person wearing the uniform on the street, they rush to him for help.

Kurosawa frequently terminates a stage of Yasumoto's learning process with a didactic monologue by Red Beard, which makes it easier for the audience to comprehend the nature of the young intern's learning process. One of the earlier examples is Red Beard's comment on corrupt officials after his and Yasumoto's visit to Lord Matsudaira, whom he has charged an exorbitant medical fee. Yasumoto discovers Red Beard's flexibility; Red Beard tells him that his unlawful conduct is simply a means of helping the poor. Thus, Red Beard emphasizes the politically bleak society in which the transcendence of the existing corrupt system is the sole means by which one can avoid victimization by that corrupt system:

> I don't like officials. They publicly impose all sorts of unlawful and cruel things upon people in the name of the public authority. . . . I am not going to close my eyes to their inhuman ways. . . . Crime for crime . . . An eye for an eye. . . . As human beings they are the worst and most ignorant. . . . I hate them.

Another example occurs at the end of the brothel scene involving Red Beard's decision to take Otoyo, a brothel chambermaid, back to the clinic. A monologue leads both Yasumoto and the audience to realize that social injustice paralyzes the poor:

> The madam, who molests this child is a hideous hag. . . . But this is indeed a miserable aspect of the social institution. That old lady is also weak and cannot live unless she torments those weaker than herself. . . . But why do children like this girl have to suffer? She is physically ill, but her mind is much worse. . . . It is infected as if it had been burned. . . .

The middle section of the second part involves Yasumoto's subsequent treatment of his first patient. Through it, he, unlike the
observer, actually experiences social evil molding little children's
personalities. Yasumoto changes: the son image gradually alters
and assumes certain traits of the father image. This section is accompanied by a reading of Yasumoto's *karte* (notes) describing
Otoyo's progressive recovery. Point-of-view shots again pervade it,
and Yasumoto's consciousness of Otoyo's eyes becomes dominant,
indicating his empathy for the patient. At the initial stage of treatment, the patient resists. From Yasumoto's point of view,
Kurosawa films Otoyo's face with glittering eyes. Yasumoto's narration on the sound track expresses his dismay at her hardened
feelings: "When I am gazed at by Otoyo, I do not know what to do,
for her eyes are full of suspicion, a strange arrogance, and mistrust
of others." On the third day of treatment, Yasumoto suddenly finds
her out of bed and scrubbing the floor. Again to emphasize
Yasumoto's awareness of her eyes, Kurosawa presents Otoyo in a
different setting. Low-key photography evokes a desolate atmosphere in the narrow corridor. Otoyo's suspicion-filled eyes loom
from darkness, clearly showing her resistance and fear.

In the subsequent scene, Yasumoto not only has developed compassion and fortitude but also finds his efforts rewarded. In response to his remark that not only Red Beard but he, too, wants to
cure her crippled heart, Otoyo suddenly breaks the bowl of gruel
he is about to serve her, and asks him if he still wants to cure her.
Here, we encounter Yasumoto's first, almost melodramatic display
of compassion. He starts picking up the broken fragments of the
bowl, saying sobbingly: "You, poor child . . . You're a good child
by nature."

The following scene starts with Otoyo's disappearance from the
clinic. Yasumoto's search for her brings him to a bridge where he
finds Otoyo begging. He follows and stops her when she comes out
of a shop with something in her hands. Otoyo, surprised, drops her
purchase; she has just bought a new bowl to replace the one she has
broken. The shattered bowl—a symbol of destruction—ironically
conveys a sense of solidarity growing between Yasumoto and his
patient. A close-up of Otoyo's face from her perspective, emphasizing the tears of which she has never before been capable, reveals her
awakening to human love.

A later conversation between Red Beard and Yasumoto indicates
a further stage of the young intern's conversion. When Red Beard
returns the notes and charts he borrowed from Yasumoto,
Yasumoto, crestfallen, admits the selfishness of his having previ-

ously refused them. Thereupon, Kurosawa presents Yasumoto's long confession, making it too easy for the audience to grasp the young intern's regret of the values to which he has hitherto adhered:

> I was no good in every respect. . . . I was so conceited and so arrogant. . . . Why on earth did I rave about my unhappiness when I was not happy? . . . Rokusuke and Sahachi died quietly without any complaining though they were so unfortunate. . . . Look at Otoyo. . . . I am happy to be ashamed of it.
>
> I am such a despicable fellow. . . . While I blamed Chigusa, I was so easily seduced by that mad woman. . . . I was bragging of my training in Nagasaki so much that I made fun of this clinic. . . . Nay, I even despised and hated you. . . . I am such a despicable fellow—arrogant and impudent. . . .

As a result of his strenuous effort in treating Otoyo, Yasumoto is attacked by a high fever. While he is asleep in bed, Kurosawa presents a memorable scene that communicates the extent of Yasumoto's conversion. It is snowing outside his room. Only the lattice windowpanes covered with the snow are light while the rest of his room is dark. Otoyo reaches out to the snow through the lattice window and picks up some of it to wet a towel to put to Yasumoto's fevered head. Her gesture—reaching out to the pure snow—symbolically conveys a sudden surge of her suppressed affection for him and thus marks the reward of his fortitude and compassion. When Yasumoto recovers, we now see the result of his changed image of Red Beard. He frankly tells Otoyo about Red Beard's greatness, emphasizing his role as his model and guide.

Before his learning process can be complete, Yasumoto also must deal with Otoyo's attachment to him and its consequences. It is again Red Beard who, with his sagacious knowledge of human psychology, explains to Yasumoto the complexity of human relationships.

Thus far, we have been shown many stages of Yasumoto's conversion in clear-cut ways, even to the extent that we feel that we have had enough. However, in order to make doubly sure of Yasumoto's immediate sense of poverty ingrained in the lowest social strata, Kurosawa adds one more episode. An entire family, who have attempted to poison themselves, is brought into the clinic. Chōbō is the only survivor. What keeps this episode from becoming boring is Kurosawa's investment of ordinary reality with a supernatural quality. A strange cry, "Chōbō," rings on the sound

track whereupon Yasumoto goes to the kitchen, from which the cry
was heard. He sees the clinic's kitchen maids, who are in deep
sympathy with Chōbō's plight, shouting down a deep well to pray
for his recovery, since they believe that "all wells lead to the bottom
of the earth and that the departing soul may be called back."[5] The
camera pans down the well. It is a deep well, and at the bottom the
silvery ripples on the surface are captured. The overall effect of the
camera work and the filmic composition is a strangely sinister atmosphere; the fearful aura of death associated with the public clinic. It
is in this nocturnal atmosphere that Yasumoto confirms that genuine compassion exists among the poor. Again as in other Kurosawa
films such as *Drunken Angel* (1948), *Rashomon* (1950), and *Dodes'*
kaden (1971), compassion appears in this film as the ethical
fortification of the poor, without which the world of poverty would
be absolutely unendurable.

However, Kurosawa implies in this film that to change society
for the better, individual compassion must be channeled into the
daring and devoted public action embodied in Red Beard. In order
to become the father image, Yasumoto first had to become himself,
that is, to discover himself. His self-discovery has been achieved as
a result of his contact with poverty wherein he realized the complexity of human motives, the evil of society, and the good of Red
Beard's humanistic values. The second part of the film ends with a
succession of shots of Yasumoto; he walks out to the yard after
learning that Chōbō will be saved. It is now dawn and the air is
cool. Yasumoto inhales deeply, and his gesture indicates the end of
his journey in search of himself and the beginning of his independent commitment to the public cause.

The final section, which is the shortest of the three, concludes
the film in a happy mood. Yasumoto is now entirely different from
what he was at the beginning of his quest. He has begun to assume
the nature of his father image, Red Beard, as witnessed by Mori's
remark: "These days you even talk like your boss." Yasumoto's
quest not only results in the spiritual gratification of serving as a
doctor for a humanitarian cause but also yields the more traditional
satisfaction of acquiring a bride, Masae—the standard reward for
the romantic hero. Through his series of confrontations with interactive human motives, Yasumoto has developed compassion. We
now witness him forgiving Chigusa for having betrayed him. In
this concluding part, the geographic location shifts from the dark,
gloomy clinic to the bright, elegant home of Yasumoto's parents,
where his wedding takes place. Red Beard opens the white *shōji*

door of the room. Thereupon, Kurosawa introduces the traditional images of the early spring. Plum blossoms are in bloom in the yard, and a nightingale sings on the sound track. This scene is a relief for us, especially after we have been accustomed to the claustrophobic interior of the clinic often captured by low-key photography. It is a clear index of Yasumoto's initiation into a new life after his groping for his moral roots.

Yasumoto is now firmly determined to follow in his father image's footsteps. At the wedding ceremony he openly declines the offer to serve on the Shogun's medical staff and decides to stay at the clinic. The final scene presents the fusion of the father and the son images in a joyous mood, as Yasumoto and Red Beard walk together to the gate of the clinic. In the earlier scene involving Yasumoto's first visit to the clinic, this gate looked gloomy and disreputable against the background of the desolate wind. But now it looks like the emblem of pride and dignity, externalizing Yasumoto's spiritual regeneration. Red Beard walks to the gate, and Yasumoto follows him. The shot predicts that Yasumoto will keep pursuing the virtues for which Red Beard stands.

In *Nihon Eiga Shisōshi* [The History of Intellectual Currents in Japanese Cinema], Satō indicates his dissatisfaction with the clear-cut good-evil allegory in *Red Beard*, declaring that other Kurosawa films go beyond this simplicity in their exploration of eroticism and violence as "a symbol of man's spasmodic, deep-rooted desire for freedom."[6] However, if Kurosawa's intention in *Red Beard* is the Horatian doctrine of "dulce et utile," rather than the production of a serious film, his creation of the two character types clearly achieves his desired effect; the film is really amusing and also accessible to the masses in his portrayal of the superhero type and his son image. At the same time the film is didactic in transmitting the importance of altruism channeled into meaningful professional action as a potential for a better society.[7]

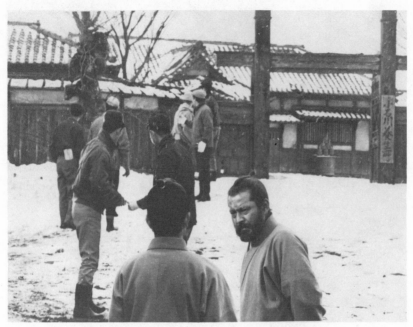

Red Beard (1965). Kurosawa in front of the set of the clinic.

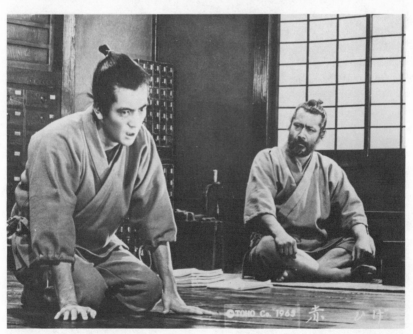

Red Beard (1965). Akahige (Toshirō Mifune) and Yasumoto (Yūji Kayama).

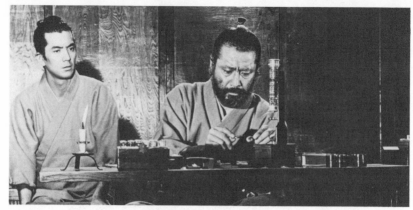

Red Beard (1965). Akahige (Toshirō Mifune) and Yasumoto (Yūji Kayama).

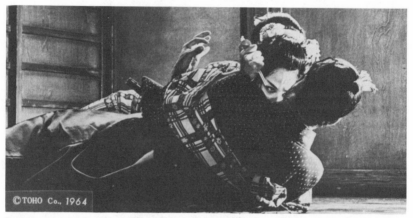

Red Beard (1965). The deranged girl (Kyōko Kagawa) and Yasumoto (Yūji Kayama).

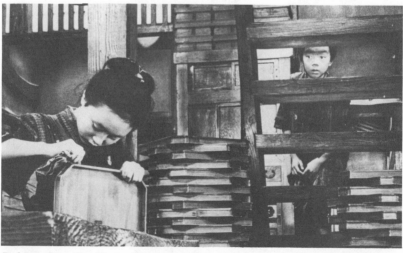

Red Beard (1965). Otoyo (Terumi Niki) and Chōbō (Yoshitaka Zushi).

NOTES

1. Donald Richie, *The Films of Akira Kurosawa* (Berkeley: University of California Press, 1970), pp. 171–83.

2. Tadao Satō, *Kurosawa Akira no Sekai* [The World of Akira Kurosawa] (Tokyo: Sanichi Shobō, 1969), pp. 250–53. Comparing Dr. Sanada with Red Beard, Satō strongly admires the spirit of protest embodied in Dr. Sanada. Though he is denied a high position as a doctor and the wealth it would bring and is not physically strong, he makes strenuous but vain efforts to make wicked gangsters human. Satō claims that whereas Red Beard's public dedication and fortitude are derived from his responsibility for farmers and townsmen as a samurai leader, Dr. Sanada's stem mainly from the Japanese struggle amid the aftermath of Japan's defeat in World War II.

3. Chieko Kotōda ed., *Sekai no Eiga Sakka: Kurosawa Akira* [Film Directors of the World: Akira Kurosawa] (Tokyo: Kinema Jumpō, 1970), 3:138.

4. Akira Kurosawa *Akuma no Yō ni Saishin ni: Tenshi no Yō ni Daitan ni* [Be Careful as the Devil: Daring as an Angel] (Tokyo: Tōhō, 1975), p. 115.

5. Richie, *The Films of Akira Kurosawa*, p. 179.

6. Ibid., p. 324.

7. Satō states that Utopia, for Kurosawa, is a society wherein human beings, freed from the bondage of social and political organizations, are united in such affection as is found among parents and their children, friends, or teachers and their disciples. A protagonist Kurosawa frequently chooses is a scientist as in *Being Quiet* [Shizuka Nari] and *The Snow* [Yuki]; a sportsman as in *Sanshiro Sugata;* or a medical doctor as in *Drunken Angel* [Yoidore Tenshi], *The Quiet Duel* [Shizukanaru Kettō], and *Red Beard* [Akahige]. He selects such a protagonist because in these professions, individuals, to a certain extent, pursue what they want to do, without obeying orders. See Satō, *Kurosawa Akira no Sekai* [The World of Akira Kurosawa] (Tokyo: Sanichi Shobō, 1969), pp. 243–44.

5

Character Types and Psychological Revelations in Ichikawa's *The Harp of Burma*

Kon Ichikawa's *The Harp of Burma* [Biruma no Tategoto, 1956] was inspired by Michio Takeyama's novel of that title, published in 1946.[1] The novelist's purpose was frankly didactic: to inspire youth, then facing the radical transformations in Japanese life, in the aftermath of the war, with hope in the future of their country. Takeyama sought to do this by referring the Japanese youth to a traditional Japanese value system, namely, the Buddhist ideal of compassion, as exemplified in his hero, Mizushima.

With a few exceptions, Ichikawa follows the novel closely, though the effect of the film is to highlight and contrast three value systems that might direct the course of Japanese life after the war. Ichikawa represents these value systems by three character types: Mizushima; a new type of soldier; and an old type of soldier. To schematize the value systems, the protagonist, Mizushima, follows heroic altruism; the new type of soldier led by a captain fresh from a music academy acts upon individualism, and the old type of soldier led by a tenacious captain acts upon collectivism. The film, like the novel, is "action-packed," yet Ichikawa's development of its purpose involves elevating conflicts of value to a psychological plane. This is the key to understanding Ichikawa's method in this film.

Donald Richie has already noticed the importance of psycho-drama in Ichikawa's work:

> The seemingly various parts of Ichikawa come into focus when one remembers that his extremely personal style, one of the most finished in contemporary Japanese cinema, is predicated upon a kind of duality.

Willing pupil of Disney, he is at the same time drawn to the dark matter of *Enjo* and *Bonchi*. Maker of official documentaries, he is also drawn to the most intimate of psychological revelations. A humanist, he is, almost consequently drawn to death and destruction. All this is somehow redeemed by beauty.[2]

The Harp of Burma definitely illustrates Ichikawa's avid concern with "psychological revelations." First, it deals with a number of stages of perception that Mizushima experiences on the way to his final epiphany. Second, it concerns the long-sought discovery of his ultimate mission that the new type of soldier reaches after various turns of event. Finally, it guarantees the audience's gradual initiation into a culminating revelation of cosmic tragedy. Furthermore, Ichikawa's specific modes of representation, especially tightly organized crosscutting and frequent close-ups, ensure their communicative effectiveness for his intention.

The film begins with an epigraph imposed on a static view of a landscape: "Blood red are the soil and peaks of Burma." A wind blows dust across the scene, suggesting a double thematic significance in this image of mobility, dust, intruding on an image of perdurability, mountain peaks. The words of the epigraph cue the viewer into a double thematic significance in what he is about to see. First, there is the Buddhist notion of this world as a world of dust, a world impure, especially when it becomes a battlefield, a world of dust reddened with bloodshed. Second, there is the actual red of the Burmese soil and mountain peaks. These offer a transition from the world as it is, to a world transformed through spiritual awakening—symbolized by the ruby, which plays an important part in the protagonist's struggle for transcendence in the latter half of the film.

The camera then focuses on a company of soldiers, led by their captain, singing:

> Autumn night that deepens
> Makes heavy the pilgrim's heart.
> Thoughts go back afar
> To the bosoms of loved ones at home.

A number of such songs are used in the film. They serve two functions. Contextually they serve as an analogue for the feelings of the individual characters. Rhetorically, they approximate the audience-character distance because the particular emotive quality of these songs helps draw the audience (steeped in Japanese tradition) into the character's predicament. Thus, the soldiers' dragging feet, marching in time with the slower tempo of the song, render precisely the weariness and fatigue of war. Yet these soldiers have not really experienced the worst horrors of war: the carnage of battle, the chaos of defeat. Their warweariness is internalized, a matter of weariness and homesickness. They are at worst soldiers waiting to confront horrors. It is important to remember that the reality of war they confront is not at all like that Ichikawa explores in *Fires on the Plain* [Nobi, 1959], which deals even with cannibalism.

These Japanese soldiers come to learn that Japan has lost the war through native villagers who betray them, after having been their protectors. It is here that the film reveals the central problem: "What is the reality of defeat? How is a soldier to come to terms with it?"

As suggested in the opening epigraph, there are basically two ways to approach this reality. There is the way of dust: acceptance of the flux of time as a necessary condition of human existence. And there is the way of the mountain peaks: a repudiation of time as a thing extrinsic to human existence viewed in another light. These are, of course, antithetical values embraced by opposing character types. "The singing company" led by the young captain accepts defeat as part of the human condition. The other group keeps resisting even after they are persuaded by Mizushima to surrender.

"The singing company" members learn of their defeat in unusually amicable circumstances. The song, "Home Sweet Home," which they sing, brings them together with the enemy British soldiers in a mutual acceptance of the futility of the war and an expectation of safe return to their respective homelands. Thus, the song reconciles them through the commonplace of hope. They hope to survive confinement in a POW camp. They also hope to work for the reconstruction of their country, each in his own way. These soldiers surrender to the British because they accept defeat as an inevitable consequence of the human condition. They accept the progression of time, seeing in its insistent turning toward the future a confirmation of the value of the individual life. When they are relocated in the POW camp later, these soldiers sing a song about the wheel of a mill. Significantly, the song's recurring image of the turning wheel expresses a natural and spontaneous feeling about the passing of time and human destiny. Thus, "the singing company" might be said to represent individual man, the character type of "humanism."

Set against this value system is that symbolized by the second group of soldiers, who repudiate the fact that they have lost the war, clinging to the past glory and grandeur of the Imperial Japan for which they have fought. Giving themselves up to the enemy is not compatible with their sense of honor. Hence, they decide to fight on to the bitter end, choosing death over survival. This fatalistic chivalry, which is not the main thrust of the film, is an outward manifestation of a kind of altruism rooted in the tradition of collective duty in service of Imperial Japan. These soldiers refuse to compromise with time; indeed, they seek to reverse its progress. To do this extraordinary thing, they must act collectively, sinking their individuality in a kind of group ideology.

Mizushima, the protagonist of the film, mediates between these two extreme views, and in the end reconciles them. Initially, he is drawn to the course of individual freedom pursued by his comrades. However, subsequent stages in his encounter with the calamity of war finally lead him to a sort of golden mean. He encompasses both life (progression of time) and death (reversal of time) by consenting to live, even as he gives his life as a sacrifice into the hands of the All-Compassionate Buddha. In other words, he denies individual life by transcending it. Thus, Mizushima represents the character type of Heroic Altruism—quite a different sort of altruism from that of the old type of soldier willing to sacrifice himself for Imperial Japan. It is also different from the commonplace humanism of "the singing company," because Mizushima embraces the way of Buddha, ultimately dedicating himself to serving the unknown soldiers, by praying for their permanent sojourn in Heaven.

The Harp of Burma is a film about spiritual quest. Stage by stage we are shown Mizushima's encounters with levels of 'reality,' and value systems that attempt to explain it. Ichikawa often lets the camera take an unusually long focus on Mizushima walking, in order to keep the quest theme predominant in the film.

Our first view of Mizushima shows a soldier's initiation into the horrors of war. The immediacy of this destruction is so terrible that Mizushima faints near the cave to which he has been sent. The color contrasts that we see are strong and stark: blackness in the landscape, and overhead a sky that seems white—a symbol of illumination. Mizushima wakes and moves from darkness into light. The meaning is obvious, though it hints of future developments. The same can be said of the background music that plays when he faints: the familiar hymn tune "Oh Sacred Head Now Wounded," foretelling his martyrdom to Buddhistic self-sacrifice.

As Mizushima walks into the light, leaving the battlefield behind, the hymn tune swells. En route to rejoin his comrades in the POW camp, he loses his civilian clothes to a thief and is forced to don the garb of a Burmese priest. This outward "conversion" suggests his gradual absorption into the way of Buddha. A villager gives him food, saying: "Burma is Burma. Burma is Buddha's country."

Next he encounters corpses scattered in the forest, and a heap of them on a riverbank. His first impulse is to start cremating them. This conflicts with his urge to rejoin his unit, which tarrying here would seriously delay. Even though Mizushima clearly follows his propensity for choosing individual, over collective, behavior, the conflict here is significant, as is Ichikawa's use of the camera to externalize his character's inner battle. Ichikawa shows us Mizushima's footprints in the shallows of the river. They meander, conveying a sense of indecision, of lingering hesitation about following the path of individualism. Even so, Mizushima clearly intends to leave the corpses unburnt; and yet, as if to keep his protagonist's conflict clearly in view at every turn, Ichikawa presents us with a deft counterclue to his intent at this stage. We see Mizushima passing from the left of the screen to the right. But when he takes the boat bound for the camp, and his comrades, we see him carried left again. For a moment, the alert viewer is confused, thinking that Mizushima has changed his mind and is going back where he originally came from to cremate the bodies after all.

We see the river in close-up. It flows on, indifferent to human transactions. Mizushima and his boat occupy a tiny spot on that flow. The symbolic association of the river with the flux of time is clear. The battle, which to men is a radical turning point in their lives, comprises only a single, insignificant moment in the scheme of time, which encompasses the entire corpus of diverse human affairs. In short, this filmic composition reveals the traditional concept of *mujō*, the mutability of human affairs, which is best illustrated in such Japanese classical works as *The Tale of the Heike* [Heike Monogatari] and *An Account of My Hut* [Hōjōki]. Thus, the picture of the protagonist crossing the river articulates the sense of futility and waste of the dehumanizing war.

The next stage of Mizushima's journey is his taking refuge in a Buddhist monastery, where he sees a group of British nurses holding a memorial service for the unknown soldiers. A medium shot of the nurses' faces is quickly transfused into a close-up of his face expressing awe and consternation. This is precisely the moment that Mizushima's prolonged conflict is finally resolved. He now realizes, with the immediacy of experience, that the enemy are also people and capable of altruism, and that altruism extends to all of the races who fought in the war. His impulse is to run back to the cloister. He comes to a stop in the middle of a corridor, which is illuminated, while the rest is enveloped in darkness. Mizushima covers his face with his hands, his head lowered. The scene is immediately succeeded by a rapid sweep of flashbacks to the previous two stages of his confrontation with death—first, with the dead as he regained consciousness on the battlefield, and second, with the face of a mummy leaning against a tree in the forest, and more corpses on the riverbank. The leitmotif, "Oh Sacred Head Now Wounded," returns louder than ever before, as if to celebrate this revelation of the universality of altruism. This movement represents the harmonious synthesis of conflicting views of life as presented in the film. The synthesis obviously is taking place in Mizushima, yet everything we see on the screen suggests that the director is inviting, if not requiring, us to realize it in ourselves. We are given no close-up of Mizushima's face; only a view of his lowered head. It is up to the viewer to synthesize all the elements of this film experience—from the most concrete flashback to the most extended use of symbolism in music and filmic texture. As if to emphasize the elegiac quality of such a moment, Ichikawa makes use of a fade-out to effect a smooth transition to the crosscut that follows.

Thus, Mizushima's determination is now clear to the audience; he will not go back to Japan. Instead, he will stay in Burma and hold services for dead soldiers. The culmination of his altruistic conduct takes place when he puts into the white wooden box (used to contain the ashes of a cremated body) the ruby, which he earlier found in the mud of the river. The sense of impurity of the secular world is symbolized by the red soil of the mountains and peaks of Burma, and is further concretized by the man-devouring war. His act of putting the red ruby into the white box suggests a catharsis, a purging of the world's dross as Mizushima approaches his commitment to heroic altruism through the way of the All-Compassionate Buddha.

Ironically, even as Mizushima is dying to the world—in a transcendental sense—his comrades are following his spiritual progress at a distance through the simple worldly act of trying to discover whether or not he has survived the battle. Ichikawa makes brilliant use of crosscutting technique to keep the two distinct value systems represented by Mizushima and his comrades predominant and also to enrich our sense of Mizushima's quest. As the captain and his men search for evidence of Mizushima's survival, our perspectives on events enlarge dramatically. We see experience in more than one version—versions that merge as readily as they diverge, thanks to Ichikawa's skillful control of the thematic terms of his story.

This is most dramatically apparent in the scene in which the captain's group encounters a Burmese priest who bears a striking resemblance to their lost comrade. It cannot be Mizushima: all the available evidence suggests that he is dead. We, as detached observers, know more than either of the two parties concerned. We know that the priest *is* Mizushima. And logically we expect this to emerge as we see his face in close-up and the expectant faces of his comrades. But we are surprised; when the soldiers call his name, Mizushima does not answer.

So much for evidence at the most obvious level. The soldiers pass now to a higher stage of truth seeking. The captain hears a beggar boy playing a harp. The tuning that the boy uses is too much like a mode that is uniquely Mizushima's. The captain's stubborn belief that the man still lives, despite all evidence to the contrary, leads to the climactic revelation of the identity of the Burmese monk.

Yet here too, another stage of truth seeking is reached. The captain sees the truth, not face to face with the living Mizishima, but in the ruby in the white box: clear evidence of the great, the unselfish commitment that Mizushima has made. The captain has arrived at the stage where he can speak to the ruby, as if he were speaking to Mizushima face to face: "Mizushima, what happened to you on that hill? I don't know . . . But I know how you feel."

A less complex film might leave us with this mesh of understandings. Ichikawa has built too much tension into his work for us to "rest easy." In lieu of simple identification with either party's predicament, we are asked to witness yet another clash between conflicting value systems. Again, the film does this by placing versions of experience in conflict. Though the captain knows that Mizushima has survived, his men have yet to learn this. As they sing "The Moon Over the Ruined Castle" [Kōjō no Tsuki], the camera crosscuts rapidly between them outside and Mizushima inside the reclining Buddha. This rapid deployment of contrasts on the screen creates a mood of detachment in the viewer. Mizushima's very human urge is to play his harp as his comrades sing; equally compelling is his need to curb this impulse. His comrades, overjoyed that Mizushima is alive, pound on a door he cannot and dare not open.

Again, while his protagonist is in spiritual agony, Ichikawa keeps his face from us—keeps us from identifying with him. Here Mizushima's face is pressed against the wall of Buddha, deep in shadow. It is as if Ichikawa required the viewer to synthesize the given clues and reach for the logic behind this suffering; to get beyond sympathy to empathy.

Thus, the director's technique again puts us at a distance, though we find ourselves emotionally drawn to the protagonist's pain. All along, we have been made anxious to see a reconciliation of the value systems that conflict so powerfully; and again, that is our reward, rather than mere identification with the psychological reality of either party. Therefore, we, who have more adequate knowledge of their situations, are compelled to remain detached observers. Our response to Mizushima's emotional turmoil will, then, be empathy rather than sympathy and we will say to ourselves: "This is how somebody like Mizushima will feel about his commitment. We understand his psychological dilemma," instead of "We can put ourselves in your position and become one with you, Mizushima, and by so doing, we share the same emotion."

"The Moon Over the Ruined Castle" sung by Mizushima's comrades has a great thematic relevance in this scene. The moon is invested with the cyclic pattern of nature, which operates on all the earthly phenomena of human creation epitomized by the castle which is now in ruins. Thus, the song reinforces *mujō*, the sense of futility and waste of all the human transactions, including the war fought by Mizushima and his comrades.

The subsequent stage of the spiritual revelation of Mizushima's comrades takes place when Mizushima comes near the barricade of their POW camp, with two parrots on his shoulder. It is precisely at this moment that they realize that their message delivered to him through one parrot, "Let's go back to Japan together, Mizushima," has not moved him. Mizushima plays, "Farewell Song" (Aogeba Tōtoshi), expressing his inability to join them and at the same time his gratitude to them, since they helped him through the ordeal of war.[3]

In this final scene we confront the final resolution of the two options, which have been in tension throughout the film. Mizushima's final commitment is to the absorption of heroic (Buddhist) altruism, which encompasses both the progression and

regression of time, while the captain and his men, who are now
going home, affirm the propriety of their commitment to individualism. These two options can be further analyzed as two different world views represented by the two parties. The world view
that Mizushima's journey reveals is presented as tragic. Refusing to
follow his initial impulse to return home, Mizushima is gradually
compelled to devote himself to the Buddhist mission. The outcome
of his choice of cosmic altruism, which is not individually rewarding, runs counter to his genuine human wish to go home with his
comrades. His choice is an affirmation of the misery in the human
situation, which, in turn, generates the question found in his letter
to his comrades: "Why does tragedy exist on this earth and why do
we have to suffer it?" To live with this tragic knowledge continu-
ously is the only spiritual gratification he derives from his acceptance of the unselfish motive.

On the other hand, the captain and his men plunge themselves
into the immediacy of their experience when they confront the
inevitable truth of the defeat of Japan. Their internalization of their
motive consequently leads to its materialization; they can go back to
Japan and assert their individual freedom, with which they will
impel themselves forward to the reconstruction of their lives in the
aftermath of the war. Thus, the final world view of their spiritual
journey is romantic in its ultimate sanctification of individualistic
humanism, which they spontaneously accept as a legitimate option.

The third cinematic movement of psychological revelation takes
place when the captain reads Mizushima's letter to his comrades. It
brings together three parties that have hitherto been involved in the
action: Mizushima; the group led by the captain; and the audience,
detached observers of all the events which befell the former two
character types. All of Mizushima's motives and actions, which
have so far been unknown to the captain and his men, are now
clarified through his personal letter. The captain reads and rereads
the letter aloud, especially these sentences: "Doubt always assails
me. Why does tragedy exist in this life?"

Next the screen is awash in shade and cloudy sky, as if to under-
score the doubt expressed in the letter and felt all around. Again,
the camera depicts for us, detached observers, a powerful drama
yielding now to a mood of carefully balanced doubt. Then, as if to
hold out a promise of intellectual poise, the screen is suffused with
the light of sun and sea. Symbols converge aplenty. The river, so
important in the film, is transformed into the sea, the sea of fertility

and the reservoir of life's forces, toward which the individual soldiers led by the captain are oriented in the future.

Significantly enough, collectivism, which has been thus far prevailed under the captain's leadership, now dissolves into individualism, foreshadowing what awaits these soldiers in Japan. The unison, "We," is now replaced by each soldier's "I." They start telling one another what they want to do upon their return to Japan. One soldier says: "I want to ride a bicycle through Ginza Street." Another replies: "I want to work in the factory where I used to work." Again, the music swells.

The film ends with the same scene with which it began. But this time, a human figure, as well as the dust blown in the wind, intrudes upon the serenity of the soil. In the recurrence of the subtitle, "Blood red are the soil and peaks of Burma . . ." we again recapitulate what has gone before, and visualize the long spiritual journey yet to come for Mizushima.

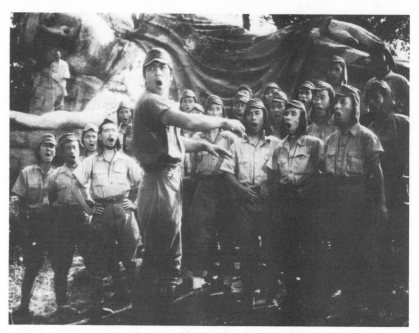

The Harp of Burma (1956). The captain (Rentarō Mikuni) and his men.

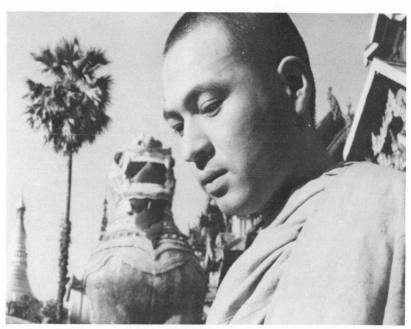

The Harp of Burma (1956). Mizushima (Shōji Yasui) in the Buddhist procession.

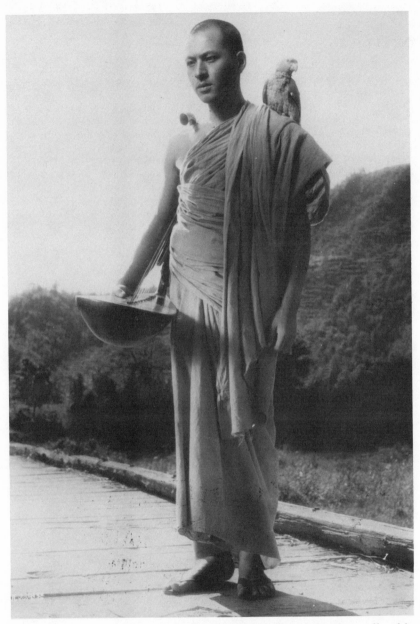

The Harp of Burma (1956). Mizushima (Shōji Yasui) bidding farewell to his comrades.

NOTES

1. Kon Ichikawa has directed a number of films based upon controversial Japanese novels; for example, *Odd Obsession* [Kagi, 1959] from Junichirō Tanizaki's *The Key* [Kagi]; *Fires on the Plain* [Nobi, 1959] from Shōhei Ōoka's novel of the same title; and *The Broken Commandment* [Hakai, 1961], taken from Tōson Shimazaki's naturalist novel of the same title. He has also made *Conflagration* [Enjō, 1958], an adaptation of Yukio Mishima's *The Temple of the Golden Pavilion* [Kinkakuji]. For a general critical introduction to Ichikawa's works, see Donald Richie, *Japanese Cinema: Film Style and National Character* (Garden City, N.Y.: Doubleday Anchor, 1971), pp. 181–97, and "The Several Sides of Kon Ichikawa," *Sight and Sound* 35 (Spring 1966): 84–86.

2. Richie, *Japanese Cinema: Film Style and National Character*, p. 196.

3. Japanese students frequently sing this song at a graduation ceremony, expressing their gratitude to their teachers.

Part 3
MOOD

6

Atmosphere and Thematic Conflict in Mizoguchi's *Ugetsu*

It has been said that the strength of Japanese film lies in its creation of mood or atmosphere by presenting characters in their setting. Kenji Mizoguchi's major films exemplify this feature of Japanese cinema. Early examples in Mizoguchi's films include the final, nocturnal scene of the bridge from *Osaka Elegy* [Naniwa Erejī, 1936], the frequent takes of the small alley from *Sisters of the Gion* [Gion no Shimai, 1936], and the moon-viewing festival scene from *Miss Oyu* [Oyūsama, 1951]. *Ugetsu* [Ugetsu Monogatari, 1953], the 1953 Venice Festival Silver Lion Prize winner, is, however, the best example of his assiduous evocation of mood. In this film Mizoguchi knows exactly how to put atmosphere to work at both thematic and stylistic levels.

The central theme of *Ugetsu* evolves around the question: "How should one come to terms with life in the midst of civil war?" This is clearly indicated in Mizoguchi's letter to Yoshikata Yoda, the screenwriter of *Ugetsu:*

> Whether war originated in the ruler's personal motive or public concern, how violence disguised as war oppresses and torments the populace both physically and spiritually! However, they have to keep living in direct confrontation with this violence. I want to emphasize this as the main theme of the film. . . .[1]

This theme is of highly realistic, political concern, and it entails two conflicting ways of confronting the war. Through the creation of mood, Mizoguchi makes sure that we see the thematic conflict at different levels of perception. He invests the harsh reality of war with mood. Through his control of the camera, mood incites or invites us to absorb ourselves right in it and feel it. Especially when mood reflects the inner reality of the individual character, it helps us to feel his predicament as our own felt experience. In other words, mood provides variation in our rhetorical stance. In *Ugetsu* we must basically remain detached observers of the opposing choices of action in adapting to the civil war, because our perspective on the individual character's action is much wider than his own. However, mood leads us to vacillate between detachment and empathy.

Furthermore, the film treats a dual reality grounded in the supernatural and the natural; the supernatural represented by the world of ghosts, and the natural most tangibly represented by a world at war. The epigraph on the screen at the onset of the film illustrates this: "Strange incidents and supernatural existence in *Tales of Moonlight and Rain* (Ugetsu Monogatari)[2] evoke in a contemporary man's mind various fantasies. This film was made in order to visualize those fantasies."

The fusion of the supernatural aura or atmosphere with realistic setting becomes increasingly dominant in the second part of the film, which focuses on Genjūrō's infatuation with the ghost, Princess Wakasa. Here, a highly stylized lyricism, provided by the supernatural mood, contrasts with the crude realism of war. Visions of integration again make us see the individual character's conflict in a more enriching way, because we oscillate between indulgence in illusion and reflection upon social reality.

Significantly, mood largely contributes to the aesthetic presentation of the thematic conflict that becomes more evident in the middle of the film. Scenes such as the boat sequence and the lawn sequence could well stand alone as proof of Mizoguchi's superb mastery of formal pattern. There Mizoguchi employs to the fullest what is considered to be the core of his style: the one-scene, one-shot method (the long take), the long shot, the dissolve, and low-key photography.

The film's action examines two ways of confronting the civil war. The first, represented by Genjūrō, Tōbei, and to a certain extent Ohama, Tōbei's wife, is the way of opportunistic greed. It ensures geographic mobility. The second, represented by Miyagi, Genjūrō's wife, is the way of optimistic endurance. It involves commitment to her community and orientation toward the future.

The first way would seem impossible, given the rigid socioeconomic structure of feudal Japan where geographic mobility was not allowed the common people, but the turmoil of the sixteenth-century civil war that shook the foundations of feudalism itself provided enough dislocation to permit it. The first part of the film concentrates on the clash of these dichotomous values and the resultant dissolution of the family. The second part shows Genjūrō's obsession with illusion and the restoration of the family.

The film opens with the epigraph, which establishes both the historical and geographic settings of the film, elements that are indispensable to the thematic conflict. The time is the end of the sixteenth-century, a time when feudal lords constantly vied with one another for military supremacy. The location is the north shore of Lake Biwa in Ōmi Province. It is very close to the capital (Kyoto) and is thus subject to the ravages of civil war at any time.

At this early stage, we already witness Mizoguchi's intricate camera work, moving slowly from the general to the particular. First, the camera captures an entire small community at the foot of the mountain. Then, it slowly travels across the field past a stand of trees, pans 360 degrees, and finally stops, displaying a potter and his wife in front of their small house. They are loading pottery onto a wagon. Suddenly, sharp reports of rifles in the distance disturb the serene atmosphere of the village. Throughout the film rifles and guns reverberate on the sound track; they constantly remind us of the fact of war as a tangible reality which the characters confront, a phenomenon distinctly opposed to the supernatural reality which they must also experience.

In the next scene, Mizoguchi lets the individual characters verbalize their choice of action in adapting to the war. Two potters— Genjūrō and his brother, Tōbei—insist on taking a wagonful of pottery to the nearest town, risking the danger of the battles raging near the village. Tōbei claims that he should become a samurai since he "is fed up with poverty." Both men are ambitious enough to captalize upon the war. They are, in fact, obsessed with money.

Next, the camera follows Genjūrō and Tōbei pushing the wagon along a mountain path until a dissolve quickly returns us to the village they had just left. The chief of the village, radiating serenity and wisdom, comments that both Genjūrō and Tōbei should know that money obtained through profiteering cannot last. Significantly, he subtly forewarns the audience of the ill fortune that will befall the brothers.

Tōbei and Genjūrō return from the town with great profits from their trade. It is here that Mizoguchi dramatically expresses the dichotomy of the two options, aided by atmosphere. A long take captures the happy mood of Genjūrō, Miyagi and his son. They gather around the hearth, enjoying the things which Genjūrō has brought back. The family is placed together in the center of the screen. The cozy, peaceful mood largely depends upon the stable camera and the visual image of the smoke from the cooking fire. Genjūrō shows Miyagi a new kimono, saying: "I wanted to buy you a kimono all these years, and at last my dream came true." His wife gratefully answers: "I rejoice in this dress but only because it expresses your love." Mizoguchi lulls us into this peaceful mood; we begin to share in this obvious contentment. Since what we see in front of us is an extension of our ordinary world—the universal, empathy is our spontaneous reaction.

However, this moment of solidarity and contentment is suddenly broken both thematically and visually when Genjūrō starts showing off his purchases. Our empathetic mood vanishes as he brags about his new wealth: "Dried fish, oil, flour and rice cakes— all bought with money. With money there is no suffering. Without money hope flies." He goes to a corner of the kitchen, leaving his wife. She silently checks the cooking pot hung over the hearth.

This visual separation marks the beginning of the dissolution of the family: it not only signifies a division between the two options (represented by husband and wife respectively) but also foreshadows the husband's choice of geographic mobility. Now Mizoguchi wants us to take the inside view of Miyagi and give her values the benefit on a sympathetic hearing. He does this by focus- ing the camera on her. The husband, now out of focus in the corner of the kitchen, indicates his intention to capitalize on the war: "War has brought us profit and a business boom." Miyagi protests: "Next time it won't do."

The subsequent scene shows a greater tension between the two options. The marriage of Genjūrō and Miyagi is to be endangered. They are now making pottery, and the irritable husband asks his wife to turn the potter's wheel faster. The little boy's cry for his mother's milk is ignored. We are now alert viewers who, with detachment, contemplate and reflect on the clash of the two value systems. Irony contributes to this rhetorical stance: the light, rhythmic music, which is in complete harmony with the rotating wheel, is in contrast with the visual dissolution of the family. Miyagi sighs, saying: "All I want is that we work together, praying to be happy together—the three of us."

In Tōbei's family, Mizoguchi presents choices of action in another light. Tōbei's strong inclination toward social mobility is parallel to Genjūrō's obsession with financial gain. Tōbei's ambition is to become a samurai, which, he thinks, will liberate him from the drudgery of the life of a farmer. When he goes to the town, Tōbei realizes that the financial power to buy a sword and a suit of armor can secure his ascent to samuraihood in the war. Tōbei, who is too poor to realize his ambition, goes home and faces his wife, who has been waiting in Genjūrō's house, worrying about him.

When Mizoguchi shifts the geographic focus of the film from the interior of Genjūrō's house to the exterior, he increases our sense of the contrast between these four persons' motives, again aided by mood. Genjūrō, Miyagi, Tōbei, and Ohama are now busy with pottery making. The bright fire from the kiln diffuses the darkness of the night surrounding the four. This meeting of light and dark intensifies the quiet nocturnal atmosphere, which could be disturbed at any time by the arrival of soldiers. Genjūrō and Tōbei's allusions to money became more frequent. Profiteering has been firmly established as chief among their ambitions. Mizoguchi proceeds to expose us to a more realistic view of the historical milieu. First, through Miyagi's speech, he expresses disapproval of Genjūrō and Tōbei's new ambition: "Is this a man's way? Up to now he [Genjūrō] has been steady. War has changed men." On the contrary, Ohama defends both men's motives, saying: "They have thrown everything into this kiln, body and soul." Then, the war itself arrives with the roar of the Shibata army approaching the village.

The villagers' fears of the ransacking army are rendered through the appropriate mood created by the combined effect of low-key photography, and many long and medium shots. Only the entrances of the houses are illuminated. All else—the rest of the houses and the street—is dim. Against this backdrop, Mizoguchi presents a series of long shots of the villagers, who scatter. Here Mizoguchi does not cut to a close-up of a single villager, because he wants to emphasize collective, not individual, fear. Furthermore, the oppressive mood articulates the villagers' relationship with their environment, and again we are drawn right into this dark texture to feel their suffering as something immediate to our experience. The villagers show their fear for their property, since the rapacity of soldiers is notorious. When one of the farmers is caught in a small storage shed by two soldiers, they drag him out to put him to work, ignoring his wife's desperate pleas. The light comes through the entrance of the shed while the rest of it is again captured in darkness. The gloomy atmosphere thus persistently encourages us to experience the villagers' fear as our own felt reality.

Significantly, throughout this sequence, Mizoguchi introduces a close-up only once and that extremely effectively. While the villagers flee toward the mountain, Miyagi rushes into the house to get her boy out of bed and holds him in her arms. Suddenly, Mizoguchi presents a close-up of her face. He thus calls our attention to her genuine love for her family, which remains intact throughout the calamity of war.

Mizoguchi keeps portraying the collective misery that war has brought to the villagers all the way through this sequence. One of the most vivid, general depictions of suffering occur toward the end of this sequence. This time Mizoguchi's camera slowly dollies along a group of villagers making their way up the mountain. First, the camera, in a long-shot take, moves with the villagers pushing a wagon up the slope. Next, in a medium shot it travels with the group crossing the mountain path and then once more it follows them reaching the summit.

After Genjūrō discovers that the pottery they fired during the attack of the Shibata army is undamaged, Genjūrō, Miyagi, their son, Tōbei and Ohama start with it across the lake in a small boat. It is here that we are introduced to a prime example of Mizoguchi's supernatural mood, so highly acclaimed by so many critics. The mood is created by four cinematic devices: the almost static camera; low-key photography; a combination of long and medium shots; and acoustic effects. Furthermore, Mizoguchi lets the natural and the supernatural interact so that we are shifted back and forth between two levels of reality.

The scene starts with a long shot of their boat emerging from the mist and approaching the camera. This in itself engenders a supernatural mood, which is also enhanced by Ohama's monotonous singing and by vibrant drumbeats in the background. The drum is intermittently interrupted by the sounds of distant rifles and guns, which echo the tangible reality of war as experienced by the passengers. The boat, turning ninety degrees, shows its side to us. At this point, Mizoguchi introduces the one-scene, one-shot method, fixing a static camera on the four sitting in the boat. As the supernatural atmosphere wanes gradually, the film takes on a realistic dimension both visually and aurally. The men in the boat, drinking sake, again begin to speak of money. Genjūrō says: "We'll be rich." Tōbei responds: "I'll buy a set of armour after we sell the pottery." On the other hand, Miyagi nibbles food in silence, her face revealing sad resignation. We are again reminded of the options in conflict.

Then, all of a sudden, the one-scene, one-shot method is dropped and the realistic texture recedes. The supernatural atmosphere reasserts itself as a point-of-view shot from the passengers' perspective reveals a strange boat approaching from the distance. The mist still hovers over the lake. Although the frame Mizoguchi uses is an open one, the effect of this dark texture is that of close framing. It steeps our senses in a kind of supernatural ambiance, and we actively experience the passengers' sense of approaching danger. The drumbeats grow louder and louder, as Ohama's singing diminishes. A long shot of the two boats almost stern to stern quickly gives way to a medium shot of both. The party of five thinks that the mysterious boat is haunted by a ghost. However, the supernatural yields to the natural again, when a man in the boat explains to them that he has been attacked by pirates. The boatman adds that the pirates will take everything, especially women. Then the camera swiftly cuts to the two women's faces in anxiety, reinforcing the image of women as war's greatest victims. The boatman is now dying. A medium shot of all concerned gathering in consternation around him, aided by the repeated sinister drumbeats, expresses their horrified apprehension of the dangers that lie ahead on their journey. Now the supernatural has completely gone; all they feel is the immediacy of war.

Throughout the film Mizoguchi uses his favorite cinematic punctuations: the dissolve and the fade. Both techniques not only show the passing of time but make a transition between two contrasting scenes much smoother, by virtue of the soft texture they create. For example, a dissolve of the boat turning back to the shore concludes the scene described above, and prepares us for what follows.

The scene cuts to the passengers back on shore. Genjūrō, Tōbei, and Ohama are ready to venture the journey on the lake once more while Miyagi is advised to stay behind with her little boy.

This scene reflects the central problem of the film in three ways. First, just as in the earlier take of husband and wife busy with the pottery, it signifies the division between the two options: opportunism and resignation. While those who stay in the boat gamble on mobility, Miyagi adheres to a more traditional value of geographic fixty. Second, crosscutting, a convenient method for rendering individual relationships, elucidates the mutual caring of husband and wife, which will be at stake in the latter part of the film. The camera first focuses on the husband, who says: "In ten days, I'll come back. . . ." Then, it shifts to the wife, who replies: "God will protect you." The camera next sweeps back to the husband and the

other passengers in the boat, and then captures all parties involved
on board and ashore. Finally, through very subtle camera work,
Mizoguchi projects his own view of the conflicting options: his
sympathies lie with the value system represented by Miyagi. After
the boat glides off the screen, Mizoguchi does not intercut between
the passengers and Miyagi. Instead, he lets the camera slowly dolly
along with her as she walks along the shore with her boy on her
back to see the party off. When she stops, the camera stops, too,
and in the subsequent long shot we see her still standing among the
tall grass watching the boat in the distance. Mizoguchi has moved
his camera as if he were compassionately watching this poor
woman's plight. He has employed no close-up for directly
transmitting her emotions to the audience. Rather, he has let us
watch her plight with him from the perspective of omnipotent,
empathetic observers. Furthermore, the complete absence of the
traveling boat from the screen conveys the sense of the irreconcil-
able chasm between the two options. A fade follows the long shot
of Miyagi, investing it with an elegiac mood that is appropriate to
her sorrow.

The second half of the film reveals Mizoguchi's pervasive evocation of mood for the dramatization of the thematic conflict. One of
the focal points is the way Mizoguchi presents Ohama as a helpless
prey of the war. We come to learn that the way of opportunism, as
taken by her, is worse than fruitless. While she is looking for her
husband, who has disappeared to buy a set of armor, she becomes
the target of the roaming samurai's lust. Their assault on her takes
place in front of the sacred goddess of mercy in a devastated temple. While the feet of the ruthless samurai, standing about in dirty
shoes, dominate the entire screen, the statue is set far off in a corner
of the hall.

This take, buttressed by low-key photography, symbolizes the
moral impotence among the populace in the face of gross social
disorder. As before, Mizoguchi projects his sympathy for woman's
plight—this time, Ohama's—with subtle camera movement. As
Ohama bursts into tears, surrounded by the lecherous samurai, the
camera swiftly cuts back to the outside of the temple as if the
director could not bear to see her raped. In turn, he presents a
close-up of Ohama's straw sandals left on the road. Mizoguchi
seems to be asking us to imagine what is happening inside the
temple. From this point on, the film dignifies Ohama's sufferings
with a sensitive and sympathetic portrayal of them. When Ohama
comes out after the samurai leave her, the *Noh* chorus vocalizes her
sorrow and indignation. Just as in Miyagi's case, the camera follows

straightforwardly, taking its cues from her motions. In the next shot, we see a fine example of Mizoguchi's employment of mood. A low-angle long shot shows Ohama standing in the door of the temple; she is looking up at the sky absentmindedly with her back to us. Her disheveled figure fits in with the desolate surrounding: the ruined temple and the gloomy sky with a waning moon. This fusion creates the despondent mood, and externalizes Ohama's emotional quandary as articulated by the *Noh* chorus. Even though a close-up of her face is absent, this typical Mizoguchi mood helps draw us into her mind. Moreover, this entire filmic composition, especially the low-angle shot, makes it appear as though Mizoguchi were looking up at Ohama, admiring her for her courage to struggle through her life; it looks as if he, the conscious eye of the camera, were saying: "Ohama, you fought against these ruthless men desperately, and though you finally had to succumb to them, I praise you for your moral courage and sympathize with your predicament."

A similar technique was used by Mizoguchi in an equally sophisticated way in *The Life of Oharu* [Saikaiu Ichidai Onna, 1952], the film that preceded *Ugetsu* (1953). It occurs when Oharu and her family are ordered to leave the capital. The camera is first immobile as they travel along the bank of a river. Then, when the party is just about to disappear from the screen, Mizoguchi's camera quickly dollies across the screen and then looks up at the party from underneath the bridge at this side of the bank. The effect is one of exquisite pity taken on the unhappy travelers.

After the rape sequence in *Ugetsu*, Mizoguchi lets us see how Ohama, who initially encouraged the opportunism of both Tōbei and Genjūrō, begins to relinquish her sense of morality. In the brothel scene, from the perspective of Tōbei, her husband, who happens to be a customer, we see Ohama haggling with her own customer for her proper share of money. The subsequent reunion of husband and wife takes the audience to the exterior. It is in this scene that we realize Ohama's genuine caring for her husband, the intrinsic quality of her femininity, unchanged despite her moral degradation. Above the sounds of the entertainment from inside the brothel, Ohama's crying becomes resonant: "How many times I thought of dying! But I thought I must see you first." Husband and wife then fall together to the ground, embracing each other. Mizoguchi's soft fade terminates this take, evoking the pathos of a husband and wife who have suffered such a painful and complex ordeal.

This final scene convinces us of Tōbei's realization that his social ascendancy has been achieved at his wife's expense. But it becomes all the more convincing only when we consider the subtle way in which Mizoguchi has repeatedly stressed the futility of Tōbei's social climbing. Tōbei has taken advantage of the war, and through good timing, he has taken the head of an enemy general and been accorded a horse and attendants. He assumes that the measure of his success proves the value of the way of opportunism.

Along with this social advancement the filmic composition shifts. In earlier parts of the film, the camera repeatedly pans down on Tōbei groveling, the butt of samurai's ridicule and the thief of a spear. In contrast, later in the film a low-angle shot is pervasively used for Tōbei as he absurdly and proudly mounts a horse, accompanied by his retainers. This radical shift in camera work ironically brings to the surface the suspicion that his climbing up the social ladder is not to be seen as "success" at all but the mere illusion created by his vanity. The suspicion is further reinforced by his bragging in the brothel. Here, he gets his comeuppance, discovering that his own wife, because of the fortune of war, is a fallen woman.

In the latter part of the film, Miyagi's way of resignation turns out to be equally futile. After presenting her husband's infatuation with Princess Wakasa at a supernatural level, Mizoguchi quickly cuts to Miyagi at home. He presents Miyagi's confrontation with death at a realistic level. Her village is attacked by a number of hungry samurai and Miyagi flees from her house. Here again we see Mizoguchi's subtle camera movement registering the woman's emotional dilemma. The camera dollies along with her running along the mountain path with her boy on her back. It stops when she starts struggling with the samurai, begging them for the little boy's sake, not to take her scraps of food. Miyagi is stabbed. When she starts struggling forward, with her son still on her back, the camera slowly moves with her. Then it again stops with her when she finally staggers on to die while behind her in the field two samurai are fighting each other for the food. Again through this camera movement Mizoguchi suggests his sympathy for her crisis. Again, no close-ups are employed, nor is any mood conveyed that corresponds to Miyag's feelings. A long shot predominates, emphasizing the environmental forces that overwhelm her.

As previously stated, the latter half of *Ugetsu* is mainly centered on Genjūrō, whose way of opportunism takes a radical turn in the middle of the film. He moves from commonplace greed to the passion of love. Accordingly, the filmic texture shifts from the matter of social realism to a supernatural lyric mood corresponding to this thematic conflict. At this turning point we see Genjūrō torn between family obligation and individual freedom. However, his conjugal affection for Miyagi gradually replaces his purely sexual attraction to Princess Wakasa. Then his discovery that Wakasa is a ghost prompts him to return to his wife.[3]

Genjūrō's first encounter with Wakasa takes place in the busy market of the town. He is surprised at her mysterious beauty; her face is made up to resemble a half-smiling *Noh* mask evoking a sense of the supernatural. A medium close-up of his face looking up at hers articulates his admiration for her beauty and foreshadows his gradual infatuation with her. However, at this stage, Genjūrō's love for Miyagi is still unchallenged. He comes to a kimono shop and looks at the wares displayed there. One white kimono, which he wants to buy for his wife, is presented in close-up, demonstrating his yearning for her. The subsequent shots portray Genjūrō's fantasy, in which Miyagi comes through the door of the shop and tries the kimono on. Japanese harp music on the sound track intensifies this happy mood in which Genjūrō indulges himself.

However, the following scene shows Genjūrō's love for his wife being put to the test. When he comes out from the shop, Wakasa's attendant calls Genjūrō and tells him that both Wakasa and his wife will guide him to their mansion to which he is supposed to deliver pottery. The supernatural aura, which is to be more fully explored later, is already here: the princess's face again resembles the female *Noh* mask, and her stride is of an unearthly lightness like that of a ghost in a *Noh* play. Mizoguchi employs an unusually long dolly shot to show the three going down the street and through the field and garden of Wakasa's mansion. This method keeps us in suspense, preparing us for the coming glimpse into the supernatural.

When they arrive at the mansion, Mizoguchi begins to reinforce our sense of the supernatural through the combined effects of long and medium shots, low-key photography, and textural contrast. After Genjūrō is guided down the long corridor and shown to a back room, there is a slow crosscutting between his room and other rooms along the corridor. First, darkness prevails, and then yields to a soft illumination as Wakasa's servants light and set candles in the other rooms. Now the cinematic action is all set for Wakasa's seduction of Genjūrō. She again comes in like a *Noh* actor appearing on the stage, with her face made up like a female *Noh* mask. Genjūrō sits between her and her aged attendant. Sinister chimes—perhaps of a bell for Buddhist prayers—are heard intermittently.

The attendant, attired in a black kimono, sits closest to the camera, showing her back to the audience. In contrast, Wakasa clad in a white kimono, is placed farthest from the camera, facing it. The imposing stature of the old attendant, like that of the alluring Wakasa, is used to block Genjūrō, as if to predict his subsequent entrapment by these women.

As Wakasa takes a drink of sake from a small wine cup, we hear the chime, and when Genjūrō drinks from the same cup, we hear it again. By this time we are convinced that the chime occurs at each stage of Genjūrō's moral quandary. We also know that drinking sake from the same sake cup symbolizes the marriage bond, and indeed, the attendant later suggests that Genjūrō marry Wakasa. After this suggestion, the princess stands up and tries to corner Genjūrō, who, in turn, rises to flee. The following long shot, enhanced by the acoustic effects of the chime, a flute, and a *koto*, presents the chase. It evokes a sinister claustrophia, finalizing Genjūrō's entrapment in Wakasa's snare. The long shot turns into a medium shot, when Genjūrō is finally captured by Wakasa and collapses to the floor with her. By presenting this final shot slightly askew, Mizoguchi suggests his silent condemnation of the lovers' illicit relationship. By this time, Mizoguchi's persistent evocation of a sense of encirclement and oppression has made us aware of some element of doom in their love.

In the following scene, the acoustic effects are fully realized in order to accent the supernatural aspect of this vignette. Wakasa sings in tune with the *samisen*: "The best of silk of choicest hue / May change and fade away, / As would my life, beloved one . . ." Her singing gradually merges with what appears to be a priest's low-toned prayer from a *Noh* play, accompanied by the sounds of a wooden drum being beaten for prayers. The camera quickly dollies from the center of the room to the corner and stops on a suit of black armor, the source of the mysterious incantation. We then learn from the princess's attendant that the voice is the spirit of Wakasa's father still haunting the mansion and that he is pleased with her betrothal. Thus, the merging songs of Wakasa and the spirit conjure up an image of death in connection with this love affair.

The subsequent sequence that presents the lovers' bathing and their repose on the lawn thematically demonstrates the culmination of Genjūrō's passion. Mizoguchi's cinematic rubric of the mood, enhanced by his elaborate camera movement and pictorial filmic composition, helps him to aestheticize this mood. Genjūrō is soaking himself in the spring while Wakasa is still ashore. Holding her hands, he says: "I have never had such a wonderful experience in my life." The camera then follows Wakasa, who momentarily leaves Genjūrō. She steps into the woods, takes off her clothes, and comes back to him. Now they share the bath, and just when they are about to embrace, Mizoguchi's camera becomes, as Joan Mellen also points out,[4] very disturbing. It quickly moves away from them along a diagonal and ends with a dissolve, as if to say that the director himself is averting his eyes from this spectacle and moral disarray. This sweeping pan is in strong contrast with the earlier slow dolly, which implied Mizoguchi's sympathy for both Ohama and Miyagi.

After the dissolve the camera dollies across the bushes of a garden with raked white sand and then moves up to show a long shot of Genjūrō and Wakasa on the lawn. The garden looks like the stone garden of Ryōanji or that of Daitokuji Temple. If Mizoguchi's intention is to let this uninhabited landscape serve as a stasis, its effect is that of a sudden illumination, a kind of shock. The garden presented for only a second is charged with significant meaning: it stands by itself, transcending all petty human affairs.

Now we see Genjūrō and Wakasa having a picnic on a blanket spread on the lawn. It is flooded by warm spring sunlight. A long shot persists. Genjūrō starts to chase her, and the couple, clad in very light silk kimonos, look like two fluttering butterflies, the symbol of spring. This take is cited by many critics as one of the most memorable examples of Mizoguchi's atmospheric rendition. However, it soon becomes tinged again with an ominous undertone when Genjūrō catches Wakasa. The camera approaches them and the next moment we see a medium shot of him kissing her and saying: "I don't care if you are a demon. I will not let you go." On the sound track, the chime sounds again, marking for us another stage of Genjūrō's moral crisis, which is further reinforced by the combination of the discordant harp music and the intermittent chime. The final shot in this scene presents Wakasa kissing Genjūrō who is lying on the lawn. A soft fade that terminates the scene again speaks for Mizoguchi, expressing his grief for those who are lost in unbridled passion.

In order to keep the two lines of argument distinct, and yet in balance, Mizoguchi frequently crosscuts between scenes depicting Genjūrō's encounters with the blandishments of the supernatural, and the more down-to-earth trials and tribulations of the other three characters. The prime example of this crosscutting is the contrast between the love scenes of the bathing and the picnic in which Genjūrō is shown discarding social conventions, and the hazards of war and scenes like that depicting Miyagi's death.

After Miyagi's death, we are shifted back to the supernatural reality of Genjūrō's final confrontation with Wakasa. A priest has discovered that Genjūrō is haunted by evil spirits. Following the priest's advice, Genjūrō has his back painted with a prayer inscription to exorcize the spirits. He goes back to the mansion to face Wakasa and her attendant. In the following scenes, the supernatural aura is evoked through a combination of low-key photography, versatile camera work, gestures of individual characters, and, to a significant extent, acoustic effects.

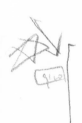

Wakasa tells Genjūrō that he must not go out, that they should move away to live together happily. While enticing him, Wakasa first corners him from the left and then from the right. Genjūrō confesses that he is married. Very low discordant music evokes the tension between the two. Genjūrō is accused by both the princess and her attendant of breaking a vow of love. He cries: "Please forgive me!" While the discordant music continues, a high-angle shot focuses on Genjūrō cornered by the two sinister-looking women, all of them in low exposure. The overall effect of these combined techniques expresses the still persistent snare, in which Genjūrō has been trapped by these women. The culmination of his attempt to free himself from them occurs when the back of Genjūrō, who is lying on the floor, is shown in close-up with the two women reproachfully looking down at the sutra painted on his back. Wakasa's face goes through a metamorphosis. Through shot-by-shot alterations, Mizoguchi gradually reveals her true identity.[5] Genjūrō must do battle with the demon who is now revealed to him. He picks up a sword lying on the floor and starts chasing the women. He extinguishes the candles and darkness prevails. Then, the supernatural atmosphere in which Genjūrō faints in the end of his battle suddenly transports us back to everyday reality. This abrupt shift in "realities" puts us in a state of shock.

Now we see only the potter Genjūrō amidst the ruins of the mansion in the grass. The police inspectors awaken him and leave with the sword, which has turned out to be a sacred relic belonging to a nearby shrine. Genjūrō, now alone, starts wandering among the ruins. He recalls Wakasa's song: "The best of silk of choicest hue/May fade away. . . ." As Joan Mellen points out,[6] the camera starts following Genjūrō diagonally as he walks away from it. This shot is counterpoised with the earlier sweeping away from Genjūrō

and Wakasa engaged in their love affair. It emphasizes his psychological transformation, his repentance over his moral degradation—
repentance of which Mizoguchi registers his approval. The fade,
which Mizoguchi has consistently employed thus far to convey the
elegiac tone, again concludes this take, stressing the omnipotent
director's pity for the pathos of the human condition. Genjūrō's
face is not facing the camera, but Mizoguchi's camera movement
has said enough about the potter's feelings.

The following scene depicts Genjūrō's return to his home. Here,
the conjugal bond between Genjūrō and Miyagi is reasserted
through his realization that the way of opportunism was the wrong
way. Genjūrō begs his wife's forgiveness. Gradually, this scene
reassumes the supernatural aura. As Audie Bock points out, the
transition from the natural to the supernatural is made in such a
way that the audience is again put in the state of shock.[7] When
Genjūrō comes home, he enters the dark, uninhabited house. He
goes out through the back door and when next the camera cuts to
the interior, we are surprised to see Miyagi sitting near the brightly
burning hearth. A fine example of Mizoguchi's evocation of mood
occurs after the husband and the child are put to sleep. The slow
camera movement and extremely low-key photography yield a mix-
ture of tenderness and eeriness: the typical Mizoguchi mood. Only
a tiny spot of light from Miyagi's candle moves from place to place
as she moves around the house, while the rest of the screen is
dominated by darkness. We next see Miyagi starting to patch her
husband's kimono, her slightly smiling face meeting the darkness.
The supernatural atmosphere completely recedes when the villagers visit Genjūrō to tell him that his wife was killed during the
war.

Mizoguchi cuts back to Tōbei and Ohama trudging home. On
the bridge near their village Tōbei tosses his sword into the river.
The implication is clear: his rejection of his social ambition.

We are now prepared for the final scene of the film, which recap-
tures the exterior of Genjūrō's house and the entire community.
The camera moves here from the particular to the general, in contrast to its movement in the opening sequence.[8]

The exterior of the potter's house, which used to be barren, is
presented first. It is now a farm that Tōbei is tilling. The camera
then follows the little boy going toward his mother's tomb and
stops as he kneels before it. Next, it pans up to, and then sweeps
across the field to show us the entire community. The movement of
the camera thus provides a moment for reflection on war and how it

has complicated the lives of the four persons and indeed the whole
village.

We have seen the conflicting "ways" finally brought to resolution
and witnessed also a complex theme worked out through the use of
mood as a rhetorical device. We have come to accept that in time of
civil war both "ways" were equally impossible to realize. The
world view that the film reveals is ironic: no matter how an individual character internalizes his motive, he cannot win. His survival is simply dependent upon chance. Miyagi's option, with
which Mizoguchi seems to sympathize most, is less rewarding than
the option chosen by either of the rest. Although, Tōbei, Genjūrō,
and Ohama have been defeated in their motives, they have survived
the war, and their very defeat has shown them the futility of their
options. This knowledge itself is their only reward as they must
transform it into a guiding principle for the future.

We have also observed in Miyagi and Ohama the prototype of
Mizoguchi's women—those who sacrifice themselves for the needs
of men and the family.[9] The supernatural realm in which Genjūrō's
conjugal relationship is finally consummated indicates the impossibility of genuine love on this earth. Only in defeat do Genjūrō and
Tōbei learn the virtue of female love, which can sustain their own
existence.

The sweeping shot of the entire village in the last scene seems to
convey a deeper philosophical idea, the concept of *mujō* (the mutability of all earthly phenomena), which must emerge from the film's
final analysis. There are two important elements that suggest this.
One is Wakasa's singing, introduced twice in the film. At the wedding Wakasa sings, "The best of silk of choicest hue/May change
and fade away,/ As would my life, beloved one,/If thou shouldst
prove untrue." Roaming around the rampart of the mansion,
Genjūrō recalls the same song. Wakasa's song invokes the
transitoriness of all human affairs, which underlies much of traditional Japanese art. Different aspects of life—interactive human
motives, love and fame—that we have witnessed are ephemeral as
symbolized by the rotating wheel. This wheel, the other important
image, is also introduced twice, aided by the director's subtle presentation of mood. In the earlier scene, which is permeated by the
cozy domestic atmosphere, both Genjūrō and Miyagi start spinning
the wheel in tune with some rather light music. In the latter scene,
which yields the serene, peaceful mood after the turmoil of the civil
war, Genjūrō alone rotates the wheel, while his deceased wife's
voice, heard on the sound track, encourages him to make good

pottery. Time, symbolized by the rotating wheel, transcends all these human affairs, whether or not they seem individually or publicly significant. In a large span of time they comprise only one insignificant spot.

At the very end of the film we see the hitherto uninhabited landscape of the field with a few farmers tilling the soil. The complete harmony of these farmers with their environment/surroundings thus evokes a sense of regeneration. The tension of the war and the possibility of coming peace in the future are thus presented as a cyclic pattern in the passage of time.

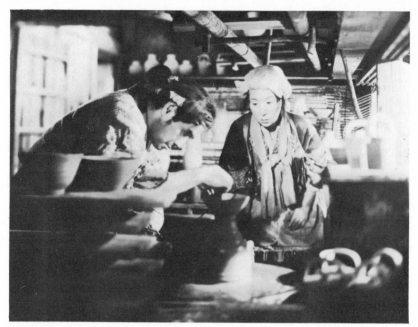

Ugetsu (1953). Genjūrō (Masayuki Mori) and Miyagi (Kinuyo Tanaka).

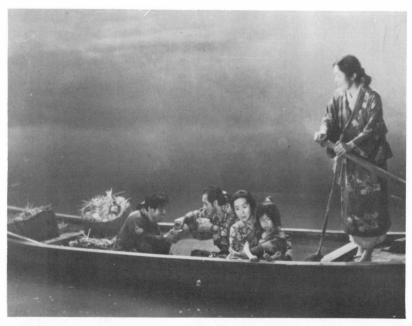

Ugetsu (1953). Ohama (Mitsuko Mito), Miyagi (Kinuyo Tanaka) with the boy, Genjūrō (Masayuki Mori), and Tōbei (Sakae Ozawa).

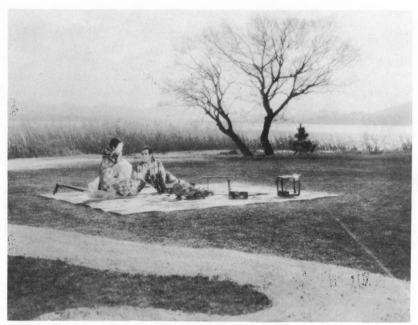

Ugetsu (1953). Princess Wakasa (Machiko Kyō) and Genjūrō (Masayuki Mori).

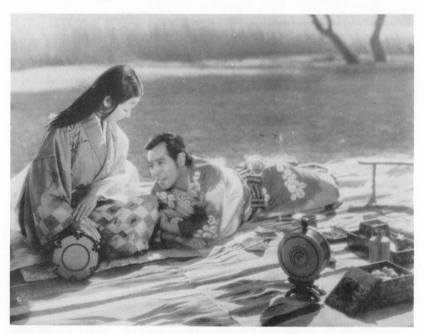

Ugetsu (1953). Princess Wakasa (Machiko Kyō) and Genjūrō (Masayuki Mori) in the memorable lawn scene.

NOTES

1. Yoshikata Yoda, *Mizoguchi Kenji no Hito to Geijutsu* [Kenji Mizoguchi: The Man and His Art] (Tokyo: Tabata Shoten, 1970), p. 216.

2. The original collection of tales was written by Akinari Ueda (1738–1809) as early as 1776 and was highly influenced by Chinese fiction, with which Ueda was familiar. The English translation of the tales is by Leon Zolbrod. See *Ugetsu Monogatari: Tales of Moonlight and Rain* (Tokyo: Tuttle, 1977). The film is based upon two tales from the collection, "Jasei no In" [The Lust of the White Serpent] and "Asajigayado" [The House amid the Thickets], Audie Bock sees another creative source of the film in a Maupassant character study, *La Décoration* [How He got the Legion of Honor]. *Japanese Film Directors* (Tokyo: Kodansha International, 1978), p. 47.

3. Audie Bock claims that Mizoguchi's presentation of the supernatural is structured around the Jo-Ha-Kyū pattern (Introduction-Development-Recapitulation) of the *Noh* play. Genjūrō's journey, his initiation into the supernatural, corresponds to the *Jo*, whereas his entire experience with Wakasa forms the *Ha*, and her revelation of her true identity constitutes the *Kyū*.

4. Joan Mellen, *The Waves at Genji's Door: Japan through Its Cinema* (New York: Pantheon, 1976), pp. 103–4. Mellen claims that Mizoguchi's traveling-away camera is associated with his moral judgment on the lovers' "selfish love."

5. Bock, *Japanese Film Directors*, p. 49.

6. Mellen, *The Waves at Genji's Door*, p. 104.

7. Bock, *Japanese Film Directors*, p. 49.

8. Donald Richie first called our critical attention to this aspect of the film. See *Japanese Cinema: Film Style and National Character* (Garden City, N.Y.: Doubleday Anchor, 1971), p. 119.

9. Kaneto Shindō, one of Japan's leading directors, who was once a screenwriter under Mizoguchi, claims that most of Mizoguchi's women, transcending the historical segments, share one unique trait—blind devotion to their men, which is unrewarded but without which the men are helpless. See *Aru Eiga Kantoku: Mizoguchi Kenji to Nihon Eiga* [A Japanese Film Director: Kenji Mizoguchi and Japanese Cinema] (Tokyo: Iwanami Shoten, 1976), pp. 43–81.

Part 4
SPATIAL
DIFFERENTIATION

7

Freedom of Imagination in Ōshima's
Death by Hanging

Nagisa Ōshima enjoyed the lion's share of critical recognition that was given to directors in the so-called *nouvelle vague* of Japanese cinema in the early 1960s for two reasons. The more sensational, if ultimately less important reason is that his work is in a genre the Japanese refer to euphemistically as "pink cinema," but which in the West would be called more uncompromisingly pornography. An example of this would be his film of 1976, *In the Realm of the Senses* [Ai no Korīda].

A more important reason why Ōshima merits critical attention is his boldly imaginative, and often challenging, use of the film for social and political comment and analysis. In a number of his films, Ōshima creates disturbing shifts in perspective as he views the seamy side of modern Japanese life. His debut as a director was made in 1959 with such a film: *A Town of Love and Hope* [Ai to Kibō no Machi], the story of a poor boy who commits a crime without any feelings of guilt and remorse. Ōshima quickly returned to this theme with two films in 1960: *A Cruel Story of Youth* [Seishun Zankoku Monogatari], and *The Sun's Burial* [Taiyō no Hakaba]. Both of these films present, with alarming candor, the spectacle of modern youth issuing violent and self-destructive challenges to society.

Even though Ōshima pays tribute to Mizoguchi as the director par excellence for realizing ideas by means of cinematography alone, he claims for himself the distinction of being the director who is best endowed with a quality Ōshima calls "dynamic belligerence."[1] He seems to be referring to his own tendency to deal explicitly with a troubling subject matter in such a way as to *demand* participation by the viewer in the director's own complex and

sometimes contradictory perspectives on events, even as the director remains (it would appear) in full control of the "outcome."

This is tantamount to saying that Ōshima is a master rhetorician
and an ideologue as well. For the critic, this means a certain amount
of puzzling out and something else as well, as we shall see: the
presence of a kind of perversity in a film like Death by Hanging,
where a marvelous shifting of perspectives and events does "work"
and does create its moments of confused confrontation that suggest
important things about Ōshima's art.

As might be expected, Ōshima's most difficult films are the ones
that are most resolutely political. They are the films that move
away from individual case history and toward direct indictments
delivered against whole societies. As early as 1959 Ōshima stated
that films of the nouvelle vague must focus on individuals doing
battle with the forces of circumstance and/or environment that
were responsible for their misery; and that such individuals must
not be presented as isolated psychopaths, mere case histories of no
more general significance for social change.[2]

Death by Hanging [Kōshikei, 1968] is such a film.[3] Made in 1968,
it deals with an actual event that occurred ten years earlier, the
murder of a Japanese schoolgirl by a young Korean boy, Rhee.

The choice of subject for Death by Hanging is itself as good as a
declaration of intent to create just such a film. The boy Rhee, as a
Korean, is, in effect, inseparable from a minority whose oppression
in Japan Ōshima considers "the Japanese original sin."

Other directors have presented aspects of this "Korean problem," notably Kirirō Urayama and Shōhei Imamura. In The Town
with the Cupola [Kyūpora no Aru Machi, 1962], Urayama describes
a close friendship that develops between a Japanese and a Korean
boy in an industrial slum. Imamura's My Second Brother [Nianchan,
1959] looks at the problem of a Korean family living in a coal-
mining town in Kyūshū. It is a story of poverty, ethnic alienation,
and destruction of the family. Unlike Ōshima, these directors do
not emphasize the issue of Korean ethnicity as highly political.

Ōshima, too, in what might be called a more "documentary"
mood, examines the plight of Koreans in Japan in films like Forgot-
ten Soldiers of the Imperial Army [Wasurerareta Kōgun, 1963], The
Tombstone of Youth [Seishun no Hi, 1964], and The Diary of Yunbogi
[Yunbogi no Nikki, 1965].

What makes Death by Hanging a radical departure from all of
these films is the way Ōshima provides the subject the full benefit
of his "dynamic belligerence." In this film, the subject of oppres-

sion is given full value: Oshima adopts a complex strategy for bringing all the resources of imagination to bear on a social evil, the Japanese authorities' treatment of Koreans living in Japan. Ōshima uses the issue as the vehicle for his view of capital punishment. This decisive instance, he thinks, shows us in unmistakable form society's misplaced confidence in brutal, and ultimately self-destructive, "correctives" that, moreover, fall most heavily on already oppressed minorities.

That in itself could make for "difficult" cinematography. Ōshima, however, goes himself one better in *Death by Hanging*. He advances an extremely complicated cinematic rhetoric to demonstrate that capital punishment is an abuse of power and a perversion of justice so extraordinary that it leads to a divestment of reality itself—of the power to live and love on genuine human terms.

Several critics have related Ōshima's political convictions to his artistic method in *Death by Hanging*. Starting with the assumption that, in his hands, "political cinema becomes an attack on Japan from within and without," Joan Mellen studies Ōshima's conscious use of allegory to make his ideology comprehensible to the audience.[4] A good deal of background for that ideology is given by Tadao Satō in *Ōshima Nagisa no Sekai* [The World of Nagisa Ōshima], in which Satō attempts a comprehensive analysis of *Death by Hanging*, with a discussion of biographical details, motifs, and structure.[5] In another work, Satō discusses the improbability of the *donnés* of the film; he argues that a hanging would not actually fail to "execute" the victim and that the officials in charge would not by any stretch of the imagination behave as they do. Satō connects the elements of improbability and farce here to show how this film explores the interface where reality and imagination meet. He is careful to point out, nevertheless, that Ōshima keeps a tight grip on the ideological perspective offered by the film.[6]

Needless to say, the director's "dynamic belligerence" in this case may be a source of confusion as well as of order, so far as the viewer is concerned. The following account of this long and complex film is aimed at resolving any especially troublesome side effect that may (or may not) cause many viewers to resist its argument at the climactic moment.

It may be useful at the outset to emphasize the existence of three distinct levels of reality in *Death by Hanging*. They are:

1. The World of Real Event (tangible reality): an actual execution of an actual malefactor taking place in "real" space and time. This is the everyday world of perception-as-usual. Even its most

troubling *donnés*—a man is hanged, but is not killed by the drop—is nevertheless an easily accounted for fact. The connecting link between this level of reality, however, is a consequence of that fact: the hanged man does not remember.

2. The World of Events Reenacted (fictional reality): since the hanging has not removed the criminal from this world, and worse, since his lapse of memory restores him to life endowed with a problematic and threatening new existence, the officials in charge move to educate him back into criminality by reenacting his crime of rape and murder. Their efforts to identify with the crime are gradually (though of course farcically all the way) more successful than they could ever be in a world of real events only. Their collective fantasizing strips away their social camouflage and, moreover, it initiates them into a vision of a Korean woman they come to share with the Korean criminal Rhee. This shared visionary continuum forms a bridge to the rather abruptly introduced third level of reality: the world as imagined by a man who belongs to a class of humans so despised that his very name Rhee is abbreviated to R, so that he may stand for all Rs—suffering Korean residents in Japan. Thus we have:

3. The World of R's Imagination: in this visionary world, which one by one the officials enter into in order to "see," the moral disorder of oppression and injustice is used to develop the idea that society divests itself of the power of love by creating what can be called "the condition R.".

Of course, all three levels of reality are woven together, the first and second dominating in the first half of the film, and the third added in the second half. Before we consider the total effect, scene by scene, it may be well to pause and prepare for the great "problem" of this film, which is rhetorical ambiguity that may leave the viewer guessing a little too hard at Ōshima's intention.

Noël Burch claims that Ōshima's films suggest "that the picture is only there to tell the story," an idea "historically foreign to the Japanese film."[7] Certainly the first half of *Death by Hanging* bears this out as we see a progress of interrogation, after the failed hanging, develop into the complex drama outlined previously. But then in the second half, Ōshima seems set on forcing us to share his conviction that "what Japan has done to Korea constitutes the biggest crime ever committed."[8]

Ōshima's methods are not crudely propagandistic. His use of the camera is subtle and powerful, yet he does create what might seem an undesirable effect of viewer resistance. It may be possible to resolve this difficulty by seeing it as part and parcel of an extremely cunning method in the picture.

The viewer's first reaction, then, might be called the doubtful pause: Surely, we think, Ōshima is merely trying to give us both inside and outside views of R. But does he really mean to force the issue so? Does he really insist that we assent to his position vis-à-vis the treatment of Koreans by Japan?

The viewer who moves to a second level of reaction will see that such is not the case; that Ōshima has deliberately set a trap for his audience. His real purpose is to "push" for rhetorical distance after all. Just as Ōshima uses levels of reality both "real" and "unreal" to prevent our simple/wholesome identifying with the story told in the picture, so too his use of the violently reductive argument keeps us at a proper distance.

To see how he does this, we must concentrate on Ōshima's use of complex patterns of spatial differentation. A section-by-section analysis is suggested by the film itself, with its Godard-like subtitle divisions using philosophical propositions like "R Refuses To Be R." Then too, there is a corresponding shift from documentary detachment to dramatic involvement—a shift expressed directly by the camera.

The film begins with a straightforward documentary question about capital punishment (an issue that looms large in contemporary Japan). We see the results of a poll taken in June 1957. Respondents were asked if they were for or against the abolition of capital punishment. The results: For, 71 percent; Against, 16 percent; Undecided, 13 percent. A question is flashed on the screen. Then, Ōshima asks: "Those who voted for abolition, have you ever seen an execution chamber or an execution?" When the two lines— "Have you seen an execution chamber?" and "Have you seen an execution?"—appear on the screen in succession, each projected for a long time, we already feel the intensity and seriousness the director brings to this central problem of the film: "Should there be capital punishment?"

Ōshima is now ready to satisfy our curiosity about the execution chamber. The news-commentator-like narrator's voice describes the prison compound, while a helicopter shot moves from the general to the particular. The camera sweeps and offers a bird's-eye view of the compound. Then it pans in on the execution chamber and moves into the interior. This mode of documentary presentation initially establishes a "neutral" perspective—the opening rhetorical stance.

Ironically, the entire prison that we see on the screen is quite unlike what we normally associate with the "gate of hell." It resembles, rather, a congenial new housing development. The narrator says as much: "There is a garden, and sometimes we see flowering cherries and azaleas according to the season." Then the ground slopes away from the central building, taking us to the execution chamber. It looks like someone's house, about the size of an average bungalow, painted a light cream color. The interior is quite bright; the walls are painted salmon pink. The narrator's voice goes on to say; "In the middle of the execution chamber there is a trapdoor. It is about three feet square. Above it hangs the noose." Following his voice, the camera first focuses on the trapdoor and then takes a close-up of the noose hanging from the ceiling. Later, after R's body falls from the trapdoor during the execution, there is another such close-up. These shots of the white noose against the black background become fixed in our mind almost as a shock: then we realize that the recurrent presentation of this image is intentional. First, the rigid, symmetrical image, illustrating the central problem of the film, enhances its abstract logic. Second, its roundness foreshadows what we experience at the end: the circular movement of that logic, starting from nowhere and reaching somewhere. It indicates the impossibility of giving any definite view on the central problem. Significantly, this wayward progression of argument is also buttressed by an appropriate method of presentation. Ōshima edits the first half of the film in such a way that each cut is disjunct, clearly separate from the others. He also uses an element of redundancy, purposely presenting the same actions twice.

The first section, "R's Body Rejected Capital Punishment," projects only the first level of reality: The World of Real Event. After the execution is completed, the police authorities find that R has simply lost consciousness and is still alive. Each official involved in the execution, in his own capacity as a specialist, sees this phenomenon in terms of the validity of the execution procedure. The argument proceeds then in legal or philosophical terms according to what each believes about capital punishment.

The administrative official of the public procurator's office contends that execution of the unconscious is not lawful. The pastor advances the theological argument that since R's soul is already in God's hands, he cannot possibly suffer reexecution. The chief of the security department suggests that the medical doctor revive R and make the execution possible. The education officer agrees that consciousness is a prerequisite to reexecution because the convict should face his execution with full consciousness of his guilt. Eventually, all the officials except the pastor accept the education officer's view. The pastor objects to bringing R to life in order to kill him.

This paradox of capital punishment brings us to the second section, "R Does Not Accept Being R." The police officials succeed in reviving R who, however, does not remember anything that happened to him before the execution. The rest of this section revolves around the police officials' reenactment of R's crime as the two "worlds" of real and fictional event meet and mingle. The prison doctor plays the role of R. Following the story accepted in R's trial, he sees a young Japanese girl riding a bicycle, and chases and rapes her. The fat education officer is cast as the girl. When the medical doctor steps down from his role, saying that acting does not incite his desire for rape, he is replaced by the chief of the security department.

The reenactment is entirely ridiculous. The characters are, of course, absurdly miscast, so that a farcical version of reality contrasts sharply with the everyday routine of the police officials' lives. The absurdity of the entire situation intensifies our sense of the illogicality of the police officials' seemingly self-sufficient conception of capital punishment. The pros and cons of capital punishment presented at the beginning of the film become more dramatic and distinct. The pastor intervenes, still arguing the invalidity of executing a soulless man: "He is no longer R. He does not have R's mind. The mind incites crime and corporal punishment is nothing but punishment to the mind. . . ." He even accuses the others of being godless. R's monotonous response—"How are you, education officer?"—increases our sense of the nonsensicality of the "official" view of capital punishment.

The third section, "R Acknowledges the Existence of R as a Stranger," continues the mixing of real and fictional worlds. As the police officials continue to reenact his crime, R is drawn into their fictional world. This is done through a process of interrogation. This way, we learn about R's rationality, family background, and history as an oppressed Korean in Japan. The action moves from the abstract to the concrete. First, the administration official from the public procurator's office reads the verdict of R's second crime: his attempt to rape a sixteen-year-old girl, who was reading a book near the water tank at her high school. The education officer tells R that he committed the crime and that he served a four-year prison term for it. He also informs R that he is a Korean. Asked by R what a Korean is, the education officer finds it dificult to say. Then, the police officials reenact R's underprivileged origins: the poor, unhappy family life; the drunken father; the battered mother.

The result of all this play acting is a peculiar detachment on the part of the viewer. The ostentatious shabbiness of R's home, accented by the walls patched all over with newspapers, repels us. The grotesque antics of the officials portraying the brutalities of family life also create a similar effect. It is a case of "the official view" of poverty and degradation being so enthusiastically put forward that it becomes unconvincing. The very eagerness of these guardians of the law to make R understand just how vile he is produces a brilliantly counterproductive result: R does not recognize himself in it at all. "What happened to R?" he asks. Worse yet, he does not even feel like being R. He says: "I may be R since you are so persistent in telling me so. However, I cannot bring myself to think so now."

Following the education officer, who is overly enthusiastic about directing the reenactment, the camera moves around. Throughout this section, the principle of stillness/movement is observed. Intermittently, the camera also focuses on the silent R surrounded by the group of police officials, thereby conveying the threat that R faces. The more enthusiastic and persuasive the police officials become, the more silent and calm R becomes. Thus, this section again also serves as a reinforcement of the absurdity of the official approach to capital punishment. Furthermore, toward the end of this section, the image of the noose hanging from the ceiling becomes obtrusive. Behind this rope the education officer accuses R of raping two girls and murdering them in cold blood. R's head is seen in the circle of the noose. Significantly, this composition intensifies the sense of R's being cornered into his inevitable execution and at the same time its roundness reinforces the wayward view on capital punishment.

The headline of the fourth section reads: "R Tries to be R." Here, the world of events reenacted, which is shared by R for the first time, gains the upper hand. We are brought face to face with the deterministic forces that led R to repress his sexuality by escaping into a world of imagination. At the beginning, every single police official participates in the reenactment of R's crime, playing the roles of R's individual family members. R's older brothers start quarreling in front of the rest of the family, while R watches calmly and indifferently. Finally, urged by the forceful education officer, R reluctantly starts playing himself and intervenes in the fight. In the meantime, R's drunken father recounts his miserable plight as an unwelcome Korean ever since his entry into Japan in 1931. R blames his father (played by the pastor) for constant drinking, telling him that his younger brothers and sisters have nothing to eat and drink. There ensues an argument between R and his father, in which his mute mother (played by the procurator) intervenes. R stands up, and the camera pans up to his face. He enters the execution chamber where the noose is still hanging from the ceiling. In the following scene, Ōshima's irony is fully realized; R squats over the death trap, holding onto the noose, as if he were using a toilet; then he starts eating the tapeworms he has excreted. The recurrent image of the appalling noose, now transformed into a balancing aid for people using the toilet, goes beyond irony to arouse disgust toward capital punishment.

We are now aware that in order to escape from the squalid reality of his family life, R must resort to imagination to transform it through wish fulfillment. His younger brothers and sisters (played by the administrative official from the public procurator's office and security officers) ask R for money to go on an excursion. In return R has them close their eyes and gives them an imaginary tour of Tokyo. For the first time we witness R smiling as he holds his little brothers' and sisters' hands. Music, which has been absent for most of the film, now fills the sound track, raising the mood to correspond to R's reverie. R's monologue goes on: "We have changed subways and arrived at Ueno now. Look, we are at the zoo. Go and see whatever animal you like. . . . Along the next street are all those splendid houses with stereo sets and refrigerators. Our house is, well, the third one from the left; it has a veranda and two stories. You are standing on the veranda, all dressed up." The little sister, then, answers: "But I'm here." R responds: "There is the other you—the other you, who is standing on the veranda." From what little Ōshima has shown us, we gather that R is happy in his imagination, that for him the line between the real R and the imaginary R is very thin indeed.

At this stage the police officials are too unimaginative to empathize with R. Thus, the education officer orders him to stop fantasizing, since fantasy is not included in the official scenario of his crime. Urged by the education officer, R leaves his house. By this time we have fully witnessed the extent of the oppression and humiliation to which R and his family have been exposed.

R is released to reenact his crime in loco. He goes out to the street. Here, Ōshima's camera becomes versatile. We see R head

for Komatsugawa High School, the scene of his first crime, followed by the police officials with the education officer acting as
narrator. We see R, in a long shot, running over a bridge toward
the camera. He stops at a small eating place to order a bowl of
shaved ice, but he does not touch it. When he is ready to leave, the
camera glides, following R's perspective, to stop on an old Korean
woman sitting immobile in another section of the eating place.
Then, it captures a boat gliding along the river, again from R's
viewpoint. After a succession of drab scenes of the dingy eatery
where we have seen the police officials gulping down the shaved
ice, this shot of the boat makes a strong impression. It is obvious
that this symmetrical, poetic shot connotes the imaginary world
into which R has become more and more absorbed until it is more
real than reality itself. But at the same time this shot contrasts the
poetic and creative quality of R's imaginary world with the prosaic
daily world of the unimaginative officials.

R now arrives at the high school and enters a completely empty
classroom. He sits alone in the chair farthest from the camera, near
the window. He is shown in a long shot that enhances his solitude.
The education officer and the others enter the classroom, all now
attired in school uniform. The education officer's narration goes on:
"It is still six o'clock. But at this early hour a man and woman are
making love at some house. Why do I have to sit alone in this place?
Something within me stirs. . . . " All of a sudden the education
officer stands up and runs, climbing toward the top of the building,
followed by the others. Ōshima's camera becomes mobile, shooting
the party first from below and then from above from diverse angles
in rapid shots. This nervous movement of the camera evokes the
feeling that we are getting closer step by step to witnessing R's first
murder. However, when R starts after the party, yelling, "It is
forbidden to climb the top of the building," we are reminded of the
absurdity of the behavior of the overly enthusiastic police officials.

After R lightheartedly climbs the stairs to the scene of the murder, we see a crosscutting between a frontal close-up of R and a
long shot of the police officials against the setting. R walks toward
the camera and approaches a high school student reading and leaning against a cistern. He takes a knife out of his pocket. The camera
examines it in close-up. A close-up of the student's surprised face
follows, to be quickly succeeded by a frontal close-up of R, giving
way to a long shot of the police officials running toward R and the
student. The camera quickly cuts to a close-up of the girl, who
says: "You're joking. . . . You can't kill me." There is another close-

up of R, who suddenly becomes conscious of his own conduct. He drops the knife and tries to choke her, as she screams as loudly as she can.

Ōshima's manipulation of these contrasting shots succeeds in manipulating the audience's point of view. At first his intention appears to draw us into the dynamic of rhetoric, which entails a shift between empathy with R and detachment from the police officials. Relying heavily on frontal close-ups of R, Ōshima appears to be asking us to confront R's emotion directly. Equally heavily depending upon long shots of the police officials, who have become more and more obsessed with farcical role playing, Ōshima seems to establish distance between us and them. However, Ōshima purposely avoids the basic rule that close-up is used to highlight emotion. In this shot, R's face remains so expressionless, so remote from us that we are discouraged from entering his mind. Even the close-ups of the victim's face and those of the knife do not really give convincing clues to R's psychological status. Furthermore, the strange juxtaposition of two levels of reality warns us against being drawn into R's mind. Thus we take an outside view of both parties.

At the end of this section, R drops his knife and tries to put his hands around the girl's neck very gently. The education officer, who has been watching R, comes running to intervene, as he has become impatient with R's inability to act quickly. The officer now, in turn, begins to play the role of R in the reenactment of the rape scene. A long shot shows him dragging the girl by the feet toward the wall of the boiler room. A medium shot shows R watching. The camera cuts back to show the education officer stripping the girl, then returns to R watching him indifferently. In a quick shift from fictional to actual reality, the education officer tells himself that he has to hide the girl's corpse because he has been observed. Suddenly returning to his official capacity as a policeman, he calls the other officials to help him remove the body. Throughout this section, the intellectual challenge of the cinematic action becomes more intense, as we see the three levels of reality shift and mingle. The police officials sometimes behave like their real selves asserting their true identities as officials in the middle of the play acting. On the other hand, R, going beyond this fictional reality, tries to escape into the world of his imagination.

The fifth section, "R Was Proven to Be a Korean," is radically different from the previous four sections in that it moves into the imaginary world of R. The officials, except for the procurator, gradually come to share R's world of imagination. As Satō also points out,[9] this new perception takes place according to their ideological flexibility; the less conservative they are, the sooner this new perception occurs in them.

Still acting R's role, the education officer becomes insanely guilt-ridden and exclaims: "I didn't intend to kill her. Oh, she is dead. Help me!" The education officer's imagination becomes overactive, showing him the corpse of the girl he has killed in his role playing. The girl's corpse is now placed in the coffin lying in the execution chamber. The education officer approaches the coffin, and a point-of-view shot (from his perspective) shows the girl inside covered with the Japanese national flag. The other officials, who are not gifted by such keen imagination as that of the education officer, cannot see the corpse, but R also can see it. Ironically, the education officer is relieved to learn that he and R now can share the same vision. The education officer takes this to mean that he is not insane. His colleagues try to convince him that he is dreaming. Then the pastor claims that he, too, can see the corpse. The prison security officers also exclaim that they can see the corpse. The procurator, who together with the doctor is still unable to see it, is annoyed, and orders them to stop the reenactment because they have already reached the core of the crime. An argument ensues between the procurator, who cannot accept the existence of R's world of imagination, and those officials who have come to share it. The procurator's argument prevails, but in vain.

All of a sudden, a woman attired in Korean costume, not the girl whom R killed, stands up in the coffin and advances toward R. From this point on, the film's action takes on another dimension: the racial issue of Koreans as an oppressed minority in Japan.

Concerning his filmmaking, Ōshima has stated: "I try to start out with the problems of the individual, and these problems should be meaningful to anybody in the world. It should not stop at the Japanese experience."[10] Thus, in the rest of this section of the film, R's problem is suddenly elevated to the consciousness of the race; R becomes a microcosmic representation of those Koreans who have been suffering under Japanese imperialism.

Still unaware of his own identity, R asks the woman whether he is really R. The woman says: "Yes, you are a Korean called R. You used to be called by the Japanese name Shizuo, but began to use R after you were awakened to nationalism." Hearing this remark, the education officer, who has all this while been eager to make R confess that he is R, is overly pleased. He pleads with the woman to cooperate so that R's execution can proceed. She rounds on him fiercely, saying: "I am against capital punishment."

Though R's encounter with the woman involves the very complex political and racial problems confronted by the two, the frequent interruptions in their dialogue by the police officials divert our critical attention from R's inner world. For example, while the pastor is watching R touch the woman, he makes fun of R, saying: "Those who look at a woman with lust have already sinned with her in their hearts." This comic touch neutralizes the otherwise tense scene. Through this strange framework of the world of imagination, in which R and the Korean woman interact and which the police officials cannot fully comprehend, Ōshima creates two different views of the Korean minority in Japan: the real view taken by the Korean woman and by R, and the less real view taken by the police officials.

When R touches the Korean woman's hand that is silently extended toward him, the camera cuts back to the pastor, who again mocks R, saying: "He who feels sexual desire has already done the deed." Then, the camera travels diagonally toward R and the woman and approaches the one-scene, one-shot method, while she talks about the suffering of Korean women: "R, you are touching the Korean's skin, which bears the long, painful history of the Korean race. When the race is sad, women especially are sad. There are no women my age from the Southern part of Korea who do not bear scars. They were beaten by their fathers or injured by their husbands, and some of them committed suicide, slitting their wrists. . . ."

Then the camera moves again diagonally this time toward the other party, who have been watching R and the woman. The administrative officer from the procurator's office adds his own view to the woman's remark: "The history of Korean people comprises a five-thousand-year occupation by other races. Especially in modern times, its cities have been ransacked and its people murdered, as victims of Japanese imperialism for thirty-six years."

The diagonal crosscutting back and forth between the two parties arouses further irritation or critical confusion, beyond what has already been generated by our confrontation with not only two levels of reality (actual reality versus R's imaginary world) but also the juxtaposition of the serious and the farcical. Our critical burden again increases when Ōshima begins a series of rapid shots showing R and the woman. When the woman tells R to put his head on her knees, Ōshima employs a medium frontal shot of both R and the woman. This is quickly succeeded by a medium shot of the pastor, who explains to the doctor what is going on. At this moment, the doctor exclaims that he can now see the woman, thereby joining in the world of imagination with the rest of his colleagues.

The camera shifts back to R and the woman. The crosscut emphasizes the dichotomy of views of R's death sentence taken by the Koreans on one hand, and the Japanese police officials (except for the pastor) on the other. At the same time Ōshima's filmic composition creates a close alignment of the woman and R, which connotes a solidarity between them. The woman's voice goes on: "R, after you graduated from junior high school, you worked for a factory and went to night school. A young Korean among the Japanese. . . ." The education officer, however, is simply concerned with R's acknowledgment of his crime as a prerequisite to his death sentence. The woman claims that R's crime should be atoned for while he is still alive. She insists that R is not what he used to be when he was eighteen years old; that he is now a fine Korean, who understands what it means to be Korean. For the procurator, who cannot yet see the world of R's imagination, the administrative officer interprets what the woman says:"She is saying that R will prove himself to be a fine man by striving for the unification and prosperity of his country and thus will atone for his crime. . . ." In response to the procurator's remark that all he cares about is the Japanese law, the woman's protest becomes more intense and provocative. It pinpoints the brutal reality of Japanese imperialism to which R's crime, according to her, must be inevitably attributed: "He did not want to be born in Japan. No Korean does. R's father was brought to Japan as a serf. You never understand how we Koreans feel. R's crime was caused by Japanese imperialism. Thus, Japan has no right whatsoever to punish R."

The doctor responds: "If we follow your logic, 600,000 Koreans living in Japan must all commit murder. If two Japanese are killed by each of these Koreans, 1,200,000 will lose their lives. . . . We can solve the population problem." The woman exclaims: "There are not enough prisons to execute the 600,000 Koreans." The chief of the security department claims that this is an execution chamber and not a place for arguing and demands that the woman be taken out.

The pastor approaches R's crime from an entirely different perspective. He holds the view that a sinful person clamors for unification, such as the reconstruction of his country, in order to conceal his sexual appetite. Thus, Ōshima has presented the synergy of the enthusiastic, serious confrontation with R's crime shown by the Koreans and the satiric, almost burlesque approach taken by the police officials.

If Ōshima's desired effect were to bring the audience into sympathy with the plight of the Koreans by pitting it against our cynical view of the police's haphazard and unheroic behavior, it would not work. But, apparently, this is not his intention. The chasm between the two different attitudes toward R's capital punishment is so broad that we feel, instead, incompetent to weigh one against the other and to judge the nature of the crime.

Given this critical ambivalence, we proceed uncomfortably to the second half of this fifth section. Here R cannot accept what the woman has said about him as an extension of his own world, no matter how hard he tries to identify himself with the image of R conceived by her. In protest, the woman raises her voice: "You mean to say you don't care about our country? When did you change your mind? You're no longer the R who is a Korean."

The camera slowly moves away from them to the pastor, who agrees with the woman. After the education officer asks her who she is, the camera again moves back to R and the woman, who is now leaning over him. She answers: "I say all this as a Korean living in Japan." She then addresses R as Ōshima mingles various point-of-view shots. The first, from the police officials' perspective, shows R and the woman together, emphasizing their involvement with each other; R is lying on the floor perpendicular to the camera and the woman is leaning over him from a sitting position. Her voice continues: "R, you are no longer R. You have lost the mind of a Korean. You're now simply a culprit! A murderer! No, you are too cowardly to commit murder. . . . The real R telephoned the police after he committed the murder as if he had been challenging all Japan." R does not respond. The camera slowly pans up and stops on her, as she becomes more and more worked up, again attributing R's crime to the oppression at work on Koreans in Japan. Here we see a close-up of her face from R's perspective. Her indignant voice rings out: "Your crime is the only way for a Korean to wreak revenge upon the Japanese. The Japanese have murdered innumerable Koreans. However, we, who belong nowhere, can only take personal revenge upon the Japanese. That revenge is murder; it's an illegal revenge, but the pride and sorrow of Korea are subsumed into this murder. R, you are the one who committed that crime, aren't you?" While she pleads with R to answer, the

camera is static on her face. Then, it suddenly turns ninety degrees, and from her line of sight, it shows a medium close-up of R
lying on the floor with his head closer to the camera. To the
woman's surprise, R says: "If what you described is represented by
R, then I'm not R at all."

These two point-of-view shots—first, the close-up of the woman
and then the medium close-up of R—again discourage our attempt
to apply the basic filmic grammar of the close-up: approximation of
distance between the character and the audience. Since the psychological separation between R and the woman is both visually and
verbally conveyed, we have to weigh her definite view of his crime
and capital punishment against his ambiguous view of them. In
other words, since our perspective is much broader than either of
theirs, each point-of view shot keeps us from identifying with
either R or the woman. When R's face is viewed from the woman's
perspective, we detach from her and refuse to accept her impression of R as ours, and vice versa.

Thus, the interaction of three levels of reality, temporal shift,
and versatile camera movement all keep us intellectually, but not
emotionally, "involved" lest we feel as if we were getting nowhere
in our attempt to make sense of the film's action.

In the very last part of the fifth section, the woman is convinced
by R's indifferent attitude that he is not R. She accuses the police
officials of stripping R of his own identity: "Go ahead and execute
R. It is Japanese imperialism that has stripped Koreans of their
racial pride. And this crude imperialism still thrives now—among
you, officials, who are nothing but tools of imperial authority."
The administrative officer from the procurator's office has now
finally come to see R's world of imagination and can hear the
woman sobbing. The procurator, even though he still cannot par-
take of the world and hence can neither see nor hear her, orders that
the invisible woman be executed. A medium shot of the noose
returns, and it is placed around the woman's neck. When the trapdoor is pushed, she falls into the pit. We are not really certain what
the director's intention is in this scene. If we interpret it simply as
an allegory of the conflict between the victimizer and the victim,
the Japanese authority and the powerless Korean minority, the
ending must certainly emphasize the oppressed Koreans' futile attempt to rebel against Japanese imperialism.

The sixth section of the film, "R Finally Becomes R," is
Ōshima's most dynamic treatment of R's imaginary world. Now
there is a clear cleavage between two levels of reality: R's imaginary

world, which is no longer accessible to any police official, and the world of actual reality in which the police officials now act free from their roleplaying. The beginning presents the police officials having a party after their execution of the woman. In the center of the screen R and the Korean woman (still alive) are lying side by side ready to embrace each other, surrounded by the officials. Throughout this section, Ōshima crosscuts between the two parties, capturing the two together from time to time. This technique again emphasizes the presence of two distinct orientations toward the central problem of the film—capital punishment. Confronting R's imagination, we begin to learn the nature of his inner world, its relationship to his conduct, and ultimately his commitment to the murder, which he feels should not be punished by death. On the other hand, his ability to reason somewhat numbed by alcohol, each police official responds to the issue of capital punishment in his own way. Significantly, each official expresses his own personal fear, frustration, and prejudice. The solemnity and seriousness, with which the world of R's imagination is presented, are in striking contrast to the merry silliness and bathos that merge to express the real world of officialdom. Therefore, the crosscutting technique also engenders a sense of R's alienation from Japanese society.

Shots of the two parties together thematically reinforce the chasm between the Koreans and the Japanese. At the same time these shots rhetorically impose an outside view upon us. The education officer, who has now lost his social mask to alcohol, dances with a sake bottle between his knees, and the pastor reveals his latent homosexuality and tries to kiss the chief of the security department. Amid this merriment, the chief of the security department expresses his personal opinion that in a civilized country capital punishment should be abolished, and then starts singing a military song. When the doctor tells the party that he is for capital punishment, the entire party grows silent. Once again, the juxtaposition of the serious and the farcical exhibited by the officials warns us against being drawn into their world and looking at it from their perspective.

When Ōshima cuts to R and the woman, he uses a medium shot or a close-up of the two, fixing his camera upon them. When it first cuts to the two, a medium shot shows R touching her, asking whether he is in a dream. When it cuts to the two for a second time after the doctor and the chief of the security department express their opinions on capital punishment, it presents R, in successive medium shots, asking again whether he is R or not. The woman responds that she is R's sister and that R is really R. But R is not convinced. Through the stable camera movement and frequent close-ups and medium shots Ōshima appears to force an inside view of the two upon us. However, the alert viewer is again warned against being trapped in the director's "fake" intention: a constant vacillation between the detached view of the police officials' world and the sympathetic view of the Koreans' world. By this time, Ōshima's defense of the oppressed Korean race, conveyed through the woman's lengthy speech, is so obvious and dogmatic that we lose our sympathy. Therefore, we still remain neutral and detached observers of the two parties involved as the film proceeds.

After Ōshima abruptly cuts back to a group of the police officials, he lets his camera stay on the doctor. For the first time, the doctor confesses his past encounters with the death sentence and his present experience with it. His confession is charged with complex, personal emotions, which Ōshima expresses tonally and visually. The doctor's voice becomes excited and tense while a medium shot of him dominates the screen, inciting in us more attention to his plight than a long shot would. He confesses that he was captured in Saigon right after the war and that he was imprisoned for three and a half years for killing Pierre, the crime he had not committed.

Shifting from his past experience to his present, the doctor reveals that he has thus far examined twenty-nine bodies, and that he craves sex after each execution, though no woman will stay with him once he starts telling her how capital punishment has been performed. When he is asked if he personally approves of capital punishment, the doctor replies positively that he is for it; that if it is abolished in Japan, he will go to Korea, the Philippines, or Saigon to work as a doctor in the death cells. There ensues a fray between him and the education officer, who cries: "Shut up! You're insane!" In the doctor's mind, the past and the present merge, and he projects his own frustration onto the screen: "Death by hanging! They told me that I would die because I had killed Pierre. I did not want to die. I was in prison for three and a half years. I have been insane for a long time. Yes, I'm insane. Nobody except a lunatic can do the job I do!"

The camera then cuts to R and the woman, delving again into R's relationship to reality. We now realize that a constant confusion of imagination and reality fills his mind until the former completely overwhelms the latter. R says to the woman: "You're now rubbing my back. When your hand rubs me down, my body starts shaking. . . . This is real, not a dream. But at the same time it seems to be a dream. Dream looks like reality and vice versa. . . ." The woman replies: "Are you confusing dreams and reality?" R explains how imagination gradually overcomes his mind until there is no difference between illusion and reality: "Imagination spreads without limitation. In imagination, I fantasize the picture of a girl with a bathing suit on. I let her refuse me, seduce me, and I even kill her. . . ." During his explanation, the camera slowly pans along the blanket covering their bodies and stops on their faces. The camera's movement seems to invite us inside R's experience and further emphasize the role that imagination plays in his mind. But our previous encounter with Ōshima's dogmatic view of the racial issue leads us to act contrarily.

When we feel we have had just about enough of R's imaginary world, we are thrust back to the burlesque world of the police officials. This crosscutting is not just comic relief: on the contrary, it leaves us emotionally more detached, slightly irritated by the officials' grotesque, farcical feast, one of Ōshima's trademarks. At least it has the merit of letting us observe R's confusion of reality and imagination objectively. Now the pastor, who has already revealed his homosexual tendency, talks about his daily dream wherein he stabs each of the police officials and, in turn, finds himself stabbed. He thus presents his subliminal fear of and guilt about the death sentences at which he has thus far assisted.

The camera again cuts back to R and the woman. This time Ōshima launches into a historical account of how the imaginary world formed in R's childhood developed into sole escape from reality. For the first time, Ōshima uses a unique montage technique, through which snapshots of R's past are briefly projected on the screen. These shots are interspersed with close-ups of R lying on the floor taken from above with a panned-down camera. The snapshots are accompanied by a dialogue between R and the woman on the sound track, reiterating the fact that R has been poor and had only dreams to live on. These snapshots gradually become larger and larger blowups, arousing the viewer's attention to R's poverty and his consequent psychological problems. Repeated shots of R's right and left profiles appear until only a part of his face with his eye fills the screen. On the sound track, his voice echoes: "I follow girls. I steal. But that excites my imagination more. . . ."

While R and the woman are lying on the *tatami* floor, R's monologue continues. The camera is stationary on them, encouraging us to be attentive to what is going on on the screen. R says: "My

imaginary scenes were all those that are warped. Maybe my imagination had already disturbed my mind. When I repeat my crime in
imagination, I feel more confident. I imagined a girl coming along
on a bicycle and raped her. . . . I would repeat this imaginary
process. One day it happened in reality. . . ." From this point on,
Oshima's camera focuses on R from different angles; sometimes it
shows a close-up of his face perpendicular to the screen, at others a
close-up of his face diagonally against the *tatami* floor. The diver-
sity of camera angles visually transmits the sense of entanglement
involving R's real and imaginary worlds. At the same time it keeps
us from assuming any set point of view of his crime. R continues to
confess:

> Isn't she coming from the left? I imagined her on the right. If she
> does not come from the right, it is neither real nor imaginary. At this
> moment I do not have any sexual desire. I just have a desire to combine
> the real and the imaginary. Let the imaginary agree with the real.
> Unless she comes from the right, I can stop. But then, I change my
> position so that she is coming from the right. Now the real and the
> imaginary are one. I am ready. I'm confident. Just as I imagined, I pull
> her down from the bike and fall down together with her. It's a dream. It
> is the same as what I do, isn't it?

A rapid, radical transition takes us suddenly from R's inner
world back to the real world of the police officials. This time the
procurator talks about his experience in executing enemy soldiers
during the war. The medical doctor starts accusing him, saying
that, he, once a war criminal, was a victim of men like the procurator. The education officer intervenes to say that the procurator's
murder and the doctor's captivity were all for the good of the
country. This is another reference to the role of Japanese imperialism in the lives of Koreans living in Japan that justifies murder of
Koreans in the form of capital punishment. Oshima's intent in
presenting the faces of the police officials is thus to prompt the
audience to arrive at a deeper meaning of the film by going beyond
the manifest content of their action and remarks.

The scene again cuts back to R and the woman who are now
lying side by side on the *tatami* floor with their legs away from the
camera. Having had a glimpse of R's inner world, we can now see
how he conceives of reality and imagination. At the same time we
begin to surmise, for the first time, who this woman is: she can be
either the product of R's imagination or somebody he encountered
in his life. The rhetorical stance required to understand R's inner
reality is not identification with R; the director's apt use of the

camera angle and crosscutting encourages us to be at the threshold of R's inner world while remaining detached observers of the interplay of his imagination and reality.

The camera focuses on R and the woman while their conversation continues. R says that the girls he killed do not seem to be real. He also mentions that he remembers meeting the woman somewhere before. The woman gets up and convinces R that he has met her. R begins to doubt again but she convinces him again that it was real that he met her. R is now almost R, and he confesses his love for her, telling her how he became so fond of her. As he describes his encounter with her, Ōshima reintroduces a snapshot montage, in order to break the monotony of his long take. This time the enlargements of her face visually convey R's acceptance of the woman as a real part of his life. However, the actual composition, which places her face asymmetrically on the right, on the left, or diagonally across the screen, creates a shaky feeling, transmitting to us R's continuing uncertainty about her existence.

While close-ups of her face are still on the screen, we listen to R's confession in which he confirms his past encounter with the woman. After a profile of the woman in tears, the scene cuts back again to the police officials, who display their own racial prejudice against Koreans in an absurdly comic way. The chief of the security departments says that those evil Koreans living in Japan had better be executed all together, since they are infected with the communism of Korea. The argument, which is ridiculous to us but serious to them, is their solution to the central problem of the film: they must murder people for the sake of their country. They enforce the death sentence and murder people in war for the welfare of the nation; thus, capital punishment and war are identical. When the officials agree that since they are personally against capital punishment, and hope for the day when it will disappear, they start toasting that day. We are in a state of shock, because of irony: what they say is contrary to what they really mean to say. In this they epitomize the establishment of Japan, which according to Ōshima, justifies any form of killing in the name of national security.

From this point on, the film shifts to R's own confession. Ōshima varies his method of presentation to explore R's inner world, this time employing a letter projected on the screen:

I've come to love my sister. I wonder why I confuse my sister with my victims. I mix them all up in my mind. When I think of some one I love dying, I suddenly realize the true meaning of death.

Maybe I killed two people. Now that I've come to like you so much, my mind is no longer merely imagination. It contains the world that others can enter because when I think about my victims who were previously so vague and misty, they now seem more real to me. Not only the victims themselves but what I did and thus what I am—this, too, I see more realistically and more objectively.

From the letter the camera cuts back to R and the woman. Here we see R coming to terms with reality. The woman exclaims, rejoicing over his rebirth: "Now for the first time you are able to face reality . . . A young Korean in Japan." Suddenly Ōshima moves the camera away to show the Japanese national flag spread in front of the two. It is his favorite symbol in films made by Ōshima after 1967: *A Treatise on Japanese Bawdy Song* [Nihon Shunka-kō, 1967], *Boy* [Shōnen, 1969], and *Ceremony* [*Gishiki*, 1971].

The national flag in both *A Treatise on Japanese Bawdy Song* and *Death by Hanging* has a black sun against a white background (both films being black and white). Concerning the symbolic implication of this flag, Ōshima has this to say:

What was it that I tried to suggest through the flag of the rising sun or that of the black rising sun? It was nothing but the revival of the Japanese nation. Of course, I had known the existence of the large system called "the nation" all along, but until 1960 there was still room for social change within that system. However, it seemed that from that time onward this large system became increasingly conspicuous in Japanese society. While the sun is full of life, the flag is something dead. But one can love what is dead or can live surrounded by it. Nay, I became overwhelmed by the thought that we could live now amidst things dead.[11]

Obviously, in this scene of *Death by Hanging*, the flag represents the Japanese nation, the absolute authority, which impinges upon R's freedom and will inevitably pass judgment upon his crime. R finally recognizes his identity, saying: "Now I can think as R. . . ." In response to the woman's remark that he can let the other R die and let the new R live on, R answers: "The other R who lived in reality killed those women. Now I can think of myself and the world."

After R recognizes the R who committed the murder as himself, Ōshima again relies upon spatial differentiation. This time he initiates us into the most poetic and surrealistic part of the film. An extreme long shot takes us to R and the woman riding a bicycle along the bank of the Arakawa. There follows a close-up of the rotating wheels of the bicycle, symbolizing the continuity of life. The rhythmic pattern of "roundness" still persists, which is counterpoised with the stationary pattern of "roundness" that Ōshima has kept emphasizing through his use of the image of the noose. The close-up of the rotating wheels thus quickly dissolves into a long shot of R and the woman rolling on the grass, and then gives way to a splash in the river. Next, we look across the river at the buildings on the far bank, the river that R saw earlier from the window of the eating place. This time, however, a boat is floating on it. Instead of looking at the river from the bank, R is now in the boat with the woman. The camera is stationary, focusing on R embracing the woman. The river reflects the sunset, another symbol of the continuity of life, and R's present location indicates his desire to fulfill this life force.

From the surrealistic ending of the sixth section, the film abruptly plunges back into the stark real world of the crime that both the police officials and R must confront. The seventh section, "R Accepts Being R for the Sake of All Rs," starts with R's remark: "I understand that I am R." As he says this, a frontal close-up of him against the Japanese national flag is projected on the screen, once more emphasizing the inevitable nature of capital punishment as "justice" done by the Japanese nation. Now that R recognizes himself as R, the procurator tries to begin the execution again. To the procurator's surprise, however, R insists that he should not be punished on the grounds that although he is surely R, he is not the R they think he is. R snatches the death warrant from the procurator and proclaims that the defendant is not he, that the old R who committed the murder is not the new R they are now confronting. R asks the pastor whether it is evil to kill people. The pastor replies that it is certainly evil, and he condemns R for not feeling guilty. R retorts: "Then, it is wrong to execute me by hanging."

There follows a debate between R and the procurator, both seen against the background of the national flag. Allegorically, the procurator here stands for the concept of the nation implied by the flag whereas R defies this concept. When the procurator replies that he is going to punish R in the name of the law of the nation, R challenges him: "What is the nation? It is an invisible entity; I don't want to be killed by an abstraction." R further states that if the procurator kills him, he will have committed a murder and consequently must be executed himself. R again insists that he is innocent, and the procurator, to everybody's surprise, lets him go, saying that as long as R thinks that he is innocent, he is free to go. R slowly advances toward the exit and stops. He quietly opens the door. Thereupon a bright white light streams in making him dizzy.

This staginess is well calculated. Until this moment, we have been confined to the intense psychological drama within narrow confines. The bright light is a welcome relief, but a shock as well. Ōshima not only lets this staginess speak for his conception of the Japanese nation but also makes this moment that of a sudden revelation for us. His view that the nation victimizes individuals is transmitted directly to us.

R now stands between the exit and the large national flag on the wall. Before the procurator's voice is heard, this composition already tells us that R must after all be executed. Now the inevitability of capital punishment for R is both visually and verbally confirmed. The procurator speaks against the background of the national flag, which dominates the screen: "R, do you understand why you stopped there? You said that the nation is invisible, but now you see it and cannot escape its existence. The nation is in your mind, and as long as it exists there, you feel guilty. Just now you realized that you should be executed."

The central problem presented at the beginning of the film thus must ultimately be subsumed into the highly complicated political issue. Hence the police officials reaffirm their initial stance that as long as the nation exists, capital punishment should be enforced in the name of law. On the other hand, R answers: "As long as there is an entity, that is to say, the nation, which tries to make me guilty, I am innocent. . . . I will courageously face a death sentence by accepting being R for the sake of all Rs." Though we cannot accept R's own logic as commonsensical, at the same time we cannot help being impressed by the logical *form* of his argument. We do recognize the deterministic forces that shaped R's existence and led him to commit murder.

Talking about a famous incident involving a Korean named Kim, Ōshima comments also on R's case:

> Kim is a boy who can contact the world outside him only through a weapon. . . . Rhee's case was much worse. He could not even hold a weapon in reality. He held it in imagination. Nay, in imagination, he went to the university and loved a beautiful woman. . . . very deeply. However, because he lived unnaturally, solely in imagination, his imagination became gradually warped until the worst imaginary act, that is, rape and murder, filled his mind. By the time he woke up from

that worse imagination, he found himself a criminal, who had committed rape and murder. How can I tell such a person to choose another way of living? No wonder we are deeply perplexed and confused.[12]

After R decides to accept capital punishment, we see again a noose tied around his neck. This image reinforces the waywardness of the logic of capital punishment, which has been explored throughout the film. When R's figure suddenly disappears the moment the trapdoor opens, we feel that nothing has been solved at the end of the film. We are just as confused and unconvinced as we were at the beginning. Taking over from the procurator's voice, thanking every staff member for his participation in the execution, the narrator's ironically adds: "Thank you, spectators, who have watched the film."

Thus, through the interaction of the three levels of reality, *Death by Hanging* has created the estrangement effect in a Brechtian sense. Nevertheless, the film remains slightly problematic; the chasm between the absurd political logic of the police officials and the remote inwardness of R's world is so wide that it sometimes defeats our enthusiasm for weighing one against the other. Furthermore, as previously stated, the lengthy discourse on the oppressed Koreans given by the anonymous woman and the pervasive use of the national flag puts too much emphasis on Ōshima's Marxist orientation. Consequently, the less alert viewer begins to suspect that this is a kind of "didactic" film. It has been earlier stated that Ōshima's intention is to let his "dynamic belligerence" provoke us to make us think. Nonetheless, we feel somewhat oversaturated by his overt attack on Japanese imperialism, and are discouraged from a more serious intellectual reflection upon capital punishment that a less "belligerent" film might have made possible.

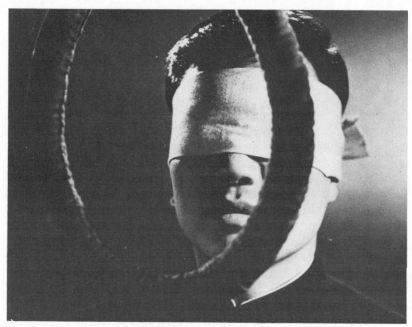

Death by Hanging (1968). R (Yundo Yun).

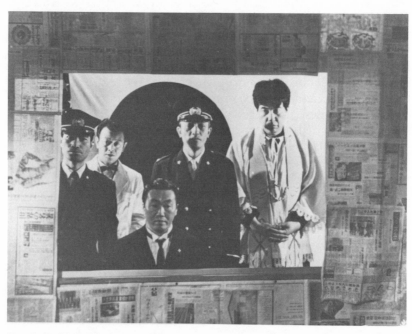

Death by Hanging (1968). The procurator (Hōsei Komatsu, center) surrounded by his staff.

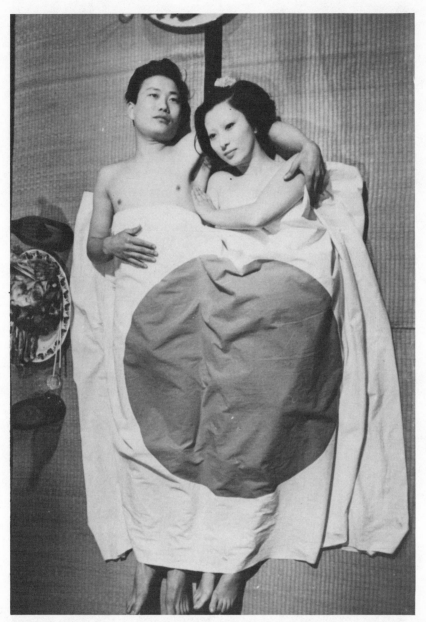

Death by Hanging (1968). R (Yundo Yun) and the mysterious woman (Akiko Koyama).

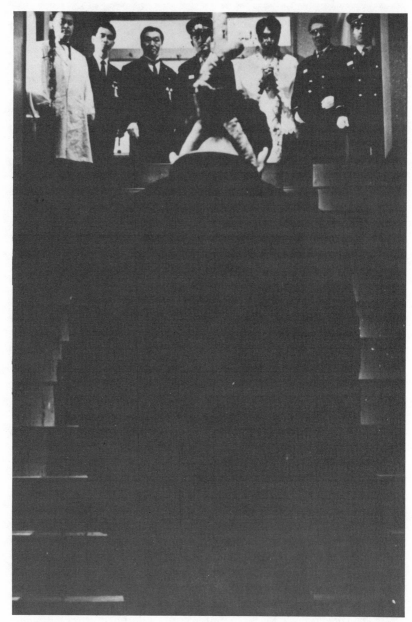

Death by Hanging (1968). The execution of R (Yundo Yun).

NOTES

1. Akira Iwasaki, "Berugamo no *Kōshikei*" [*Death by Hanging* at Bergamo] in *Sekai no Eiga Sakka: Ōshima Nagisa* [Film Directors of the World: Nagisa Ōshima] (Tokyo: Kinema Jumpō, 1970), 6:58.

2. Nobuo Chiba; Kenji Iwamoto; Hajime Nagasaki; and Kikuo Iwamoto, *Sekai no Eiga Sakka: Nihon Eigashi* [Film Directors of the World: History of Japanese Cinema], (Tokyo: Kinema Jumpō, 1976), 31:220.

3. Ōshima does not like this film labeled a political film, though he acknowledges his orientation to political issues as revealed in it. See Joan Mellen, *Voices from the Japanese Cinema* (New York: Liveright, 1975), p. 257.

4. Joan Mellen, *The Waves at Genji's Door: Japan Through Its Cinema* (New York: Pantheon, 1976), p. 420.

5. Tadao Satō, *Ōshima Nagisa no Sekai* [The World of Nagisa Ōshima] (Tokyo: Tsukuma Shobō, 1973), pp. 230–40.

6. Tadao Satō, *Gendai Nihon Eiga* [Contemporary Japanese Films] (Tokyo: Hyōronsha, 1976), 1:208–9.

7. Nöel Burch, *To the Distant Observer: Form and Meaning in the Japanese Cinema* (Berkeley: University of California Press, 1979), p. 328.

8. Quoted in *Voices from the Japanese Cinema*, p. 255.

9. Satō, *Ōshima Nagisa no Sekai* [The World of Nagisa Ōshima], p. 234.

10. Mellen, *Voices from the Japanese Cinema*, p. 264.

11. *Sekai no Eiga Sakka: Ōshima Nagisa* [Film Directors of the World: Nagisa Ōshima], p. 58.

12. Nagisa Ōshima, *Kaitai to Funshutsu* [Dismantlement and Eruption] (Tokyo: Haga Shoten, 1975), pp. 193–94.

8

The Phantasmagorical World of Kurosawa's *Throne of Blood*

Kurosawa's *The Throne of Blood* [*Kumonosujō*, 1957], inspired by Shakespeare's Macbeth, has been widely discussed by Western film critics, who bring two basically different assumptions to the film. Those critics who consider it a screen adaptation of Shakespeare's play, contrast and compare the two. J. Blumenthal, for example, in his pioneer essay, "Macbeth into *Throne of Blood*,"[1] discusses Kurosawa's departure from the Shakespeare original, defending the cinematic brilliance of Kurosawa's characterization and use of imagery. Charles Bazerman shows how the director departs from Shakespeare's text in order to exhibit a kind of control over time through the duration and pacing of shots, and through a carefully rhythmical presentation of images.[2]

Other critics who treat the film as independent of the Shakespearean original are more enthusiastic about exploring its intrinsic qualities. Marsha Kinder, in her essay, "*Throne of Blood:* A Morality Dance,"[3] analyzes Kurosawa's use of visual polarities in developing the protagonist's moral conflict. Roger Manvell's study, "Akira Kurosawa's *Macbeth, The Castle of the Spider's Web*,"[4] claims that the film is "a transmutation, a distillation of the Macbeth theme, not an adaptation," and stresses Kurosawa's interest in *Noh* drama, as indicated in an interview with Kurosawa that Satō, a Japanese critic, undertook on Manvell's behalf.

The influence of *Noh* drama on *The Throne of Blood* has also been studied by Donald Richie, whose work remains the most comprehensive on the film to date. Richie is especially well qualified to discuss the essential Japanese character of the film. His perspective is closest to that of Japanese critics and audiences who see a world view and formalistic *Noh* elements as among the film's most salient features.[5] For example, Satō cites the individual characters' choreography as one of the *Noh* elements found in this film. He declares it to be "the prescribed pattern of the movement found in *Noh*," to which the characters submit themselves instead of creating their own movement voluntarily.[6]

One of the unique aspects of *The Throne of Blood* is the way Kurosawa juxtaposes the phantasmagorical reality with the tangible reality of civil war. The phantasmagorical world presented in the film is strikingly more stylized and aestheticized than the ghostly world presented in such films as the *Kaidan* [Ghost Tales] series. Acknowledging Richie's perception as a key issue in *The Throne of Blood*, this study concentrates on Kurosawa's rendition of the phantasmagorical reality and tries to show how it contributes to the thematic unity of the film.

Kurosawa's conception of reality, as revealed in this film, is more deeply steeped in *Noh* than in any Western theatrical tradition. One way in which *Noh* drama is classified is according to the level of reality presented in an individual play. In *gendai*, or "contemporary" *Noh*, only the tangible, "real" world is presented. In *mugen*, or "phantom *Noh* drama," reality is more complex: a twofold reality of natural and supernatural. Kurosawa makes use of the latter.

In the basic plot of most phantom *Noh* dramas, the play begins with the deuteragonist, usually a traveling priest. Toward the end of his journey the priest encounters the protagonist in the guise of a local inhabitant, who tells him some story related to the locality. After he leaves, the priest falls asleep. The second part of the play is set in the supernatural reality of his visionary dream. In it, the priest sees the protagonist in his real identity. Because of the sin the protagonist committed during his life, he is unable to find rest in Buddha's paradise. He must haunt the earth as a ghost until, in the presence of this priest, he reenacts his sin and in doing so can be redeemed. This being accomplished, the play concludes with the protagonist's ecstatic dance, expressive of his soul's release from its long torment.[7] The chorus sometimes tells us that soon it will be dawn and that the priest will then wake up from his dream.

It is easy to see how Kurosawa's interest in the phantom *Noh* drama could lead to interesting developments in a film whose starting point is a play like *Macbeth*. *Seven Samurai* [Shichinin no Samurai, 1954], *The Hidden Fortress* [Kakushi Toride no San-Akunin, 1958], and *The Throne of Blood* (1957) are all set in the civil war period (the sixteenth century). Whereas the first two dynamically explore man's choice of action in the fragmented world, *The Throne of Blood* is more concerned with the moral exposition of the

central problem of man's inner nature. As is clearly established in
the opening choral incantation, "Now as in the past, unchangeable
is the path of bloodshed," *The Throne of Blood* unfolds the process of
the protagonist Washizu's commitment to evil. Shifting from its
initial portrayal of the conflict of good and evil, the cinematic action
powerfully reveals how a man lets ambition lead him by degrees to
a total commitment to evil.

In the film three important scenes are permeated by the phantasmagorical reality; the first is the eerie woodland in which Washizu
and Miki encounter an old witch. The second is the banquet scene
in which Washizu sees Miki's ghost sitting at one of the empty
seats. The final scene returns to another woodland scene where
Washizu alone confronts the witch to ask for a prophecy of his
future. The first of these scenes displays two characteristic props of
the *Noh* play *Kurozuka* [Black Mound][8], a thatched hut and a spinning wheel. The second scene offers a *kyōgen* dance as a prelude to
the appearance of Miki's ghost.[9] The witch's face is also made to
resemble the demon *Noh* mask called *yamauba* [the mountain witch].
Kurosawa lets each scene augment a sense of Washizu's entrapment
and work its way toward the final dramatization of the hero's downfall.

Kurosawa's creation of the phantasmagorical reality is, then, thematically efficacious in two respects. First, contrary to the tangible
reality of civil war, it dramatizes the inexplicable workings of the
human psyche in Washizu. Sometimes it makes us observe his
moral conflict objectively and at other times it makes us feel his
commitment to evil as our own immediate experience. The other
function of the phantasmagorical reality is to suggest the inevitability of fate and thus to make Washizu's motives seem rather ambivalent. This ambivalence, in turn, increases our intellectual
involvement and brings us face to face with this crucial question:
"Is the man who commits himself to evil merely unlucky, the plaything of deceitful destiny? Or does it lie in man's power freely to
choose evil—evil on the heroic scale?"

The Throne of Blood opens with a presentation of mist drifting over
a barren landscape as the camera slowly pans along it. On the
sound track a choral incantation describes the scene. It tells us that
these castle ruins, once so glorious and proud, show that in the
past, as now, this way lies *shura*, the path of bloodshed. The camera
passes a number of headstones, moving diagonally across to read
the post stone inscription: Kumonosujō [The Castle of the Spider's
Web]. As Donald Richie suggests, the opening scene, both visually

and acoustically intensifies the scene of *mujō* (the mutability of all the earthly phenomena), the traditional Japanese view of life that is most strongly expressed by the opening passage of *The Tale of the Heike*.[10] At the same time, both the acoustic and visual elements—the low chorus reminding us of the Buddhist sutra incantation and the hazy atmosphere—make us feel submerged in a world of myth or illusion. This feeling is sustained until we are finally called back to reality by the final chorus at the very end of the film.

After a dissolve, a cinematic punctuation frequently used in a Kurosawa opening scene, the glorious castle of the past emerges from out of the mist and takes us back to sixteenth-century Japan in a period of civil war. The following scene is very brief, rhythmically accented by a succession of messengers bringing the lord of the castle news of the battle. Then, Kurosawa brings us into the phantasmagorical world for the first time. He cuts to a woodland scene, saturated with rain and obscured by thick mist. Washizu and Miki gallop past, threatened by a thunderstorm, as the camera sweeps over them. After a fade indicating a lapse of time, they continue riding through the forest. Here, as elsewhere in the film, Kurosawa uses sounds from the natural world—the neighing of horses, the twittering of birds—to convey a sense of the characters' subliminal fear of what awaits them. The horses' neighing echoes through the dark forest, and this lends a supernatural aura to the scene. Kurosawa repeats a reverse-angle shot to present Washizu and Miki galloping. The two generals disappear into the misty forest, turning away from the camera, then emerge from it, moving toward the camera. After a series of these shots, we get the impression somehow that they have returned to the very same place from which they departed. Thus, the sense of roaming or circling into which we are visually drawn affirms the sense of Washizu's entrapment in his own fate that is dramatized in the subsequent scene.

Hoarse laughter rises from within the forest and a flash of lightning flickers through the branches. Washizu shoots arrows into the trees, thinking that the evil spirit lives in the forest. Here, Kurosawa presents the woods as an animate object just like a human being; it vibrates, becomes silent, breathes, and threatens. When the scene cuts to the middle of the woods, we see a strangely illuminated hut. It is here that we face the phantasmagorical reality together with Washizu and Miki. Inside the hut, an old hag is seated at a spinning wheel, keeping time with its motions by singing an eerie and monotonous tune. As the mist drifts in, we begin

to wonder who she is. However, as her chanting ends, we surmise
that she is a seer who can penetrate into the mystery of human
affairs. Her chant explains the futility of human transactions, in-
forming us that life is like a flower, but that it is futile and stupid of
the samurai to fret themselves with greed and lust. There is crosscutting between the old hag and Washizu, foretelling their close
connection. The camera then comes to rest on Washizu and Miki as
they watch her spinning at the wheel.

The spinning wheel, like the labyrinthine forest and the spider's
web of Kumonosujō, is a symbol of the complicated trap that fate
has laid for Washizu and which he will not escape. Moreover, the
forest tinged with phantasmagoria externalizes his moral dilemma
at this stage—the dichotomy of his subconscious ambition for military ascendency and his rational urge to curb that ambition.
Through the phantasmagorical world Kurosawa leads us to see into
the inner nature of the protagonist, just as Conrad lets us glimpse
the abysmal depths of the human mind in *Heart of Darkness*. Satō
claims that individual characters' gazing into space against a desolate setting in such films as *Rashomon* and *The Throne of Blood* is
usually a self-reflective gesture.[11] When Washizu's eyes avoid the
camera, this can be taken as a sign of his confrontation with the
dark side of his mind. Together with him, we, the audience, confront what lies there in the depths. The witch says it: "You are
afraid of looking into the depths of your mind."

The ensuing filmic composition visually exhibits what lurks in
Washizu's mind. The witch is sandwiched between Miki and
Washizu. Marsha Kinder points out that this composition
foreshadows the witch's eventual role in alienating the two generals
from one another.[12] However, this alignment also represents the
poles of good and evil, which will be represented by Miki and
Washizu. Miki's consistent loyalty and Washizu's subsequent
treachery are visually foretold when the two emerge from the forest
for audience with their lord. As Donald Richie points out, Miki's
banner bears a white rabbit, a traditional Japanese symbol of fertility, whereas Washizu's bears a sinister black centipede, a traditional Japanese symbol of evil spirits.[13]

After the prophecy, the witch disappears like a phantom. In the
following scene Kurosawa presents a long shot of Washizu and
Miki roaming through the forest. They come upon one pile of
corpses and then another. These suggest the futility of Washizu's
ambition and its inevitably self-destructional force as well. The

scene ends with a succession of low-key shots of the two generals riding into fog and reemerging from it, thus recapitulating the sense of wandering. Again, this foreshadows Washizu's eventual loss of rationality and entrapment in evil. As Washizu and Miki finally emerge from the murky forest, we feel as if we have stepped into and out of the depths of the protagonist's mind.

If the eerie wood can be taken as the objectification of Washizu's confrontation with the evil lurking in his mind, his energetic fight against the wood and its central element, the witch, symbolizes the moral conflict within him. His safe emergence from the forest then signifies the temporary victory of his conscience over evil. The controlled equipoise between the static and the dynamic also enhances the dichotomy of this moral issue. A prime example of this is the lightning against which Washizu shoots arrows versus the mist which obscures his vision. Another is the figure of Washizu dynamically galloping through the forest versus the figure of Washizu intensely gazing at the witch. If the static represents Washizu's evil inclination, the dynamic stands for his reason's challenge to it.

The second important scene of the phantasmagorical world takes place in the banquet scene immediately after Miki leaves for Washizu's castle, to be murdered en route. The mysterious aura evoked by Miki's white horse running wild in his yard, presented in the prior scene, paves the way for a smooth transition to the phantasmagorical reality. Kurosawa has thus far shown us that Washizu's initial moral wavering quickly succumbed to his ambition through his betrayal of the lord and Miki. Here in the banquet scene, Kurosawa makes us see the chaotic state of Washizu's mind clearly, through his sustained concern for the equipoise between the static and the dynamic, the orderly and the disorderly, and the controlled and the uncontrolled. It is the phantasmagorical world that intensifies the clarity of these polarities.

The banquet scene opens with a severely symmetrical view of the hall. Wooden floorboards run in vertical stripes perpendicular to the camera frame, encountering vertical stripes on a wall interrupted by thick, white broken horizontal lines. Kurosawa cuts repeatedly from one group of lords sitting in a straight line almost perpendicular to the camera across to another group sitting opposite. Moreover, the hall is very sparsely decorated, like the *Noh* stage to enhance this rigid symmetry. The harmonious composition is so delicately balanced that we fear it is about to be broken at any moment. This tenuous compositional balance ironically represents the charade of Washizu's political and inner stability, just as later on, his actions reveal his raving madness.

The old man, who, like the witch, serves as a seer looking into the mysterious depths of the human mind, quietly steps a *kyōgen* dance to the song:

> All of you wicked. Listen while
> I tell you of a man, vain,
> Sinful, vile—
> Who, though ambitious, insolent
> Could not escape his punishment.[14]

This song obviously predicts Washizu's demise.

Donald Richie comments on Kurosawa's employment of the *kyōgen* dance for moral exploration:

> Thus this entertainment becomes comment. The past warriors—the ghosts, which the witch raises—all have had the same career as Washizu, and he will end as they have. The chorus at beginning and end, the battles during the first scenes and the last, the two views of the ruins of the castle—all of this suggests repetition and the same actions endlessly, mechanically repeating themselves.[15]

While the old man's dance continues in front of Washizu, the camera pans on the horizontal to show two empty seats in the hall, indicating the absence of Miki and his son. Then it cuts to a medium shot of Washizu on the dais and then to a medium shot of his wife, Asaji, on another dais, to suggest their involvement in Miki's assassination. Their faces and posture, undercutting their dignity and calm, invite us to take note of their internal turmoil and tension that are held superbly under control. Their vacant eyes staring into space, as Satō notes, again urge us to reflect on their inner reality together with them. Washizu tells the old man to stop dancing. From this point the action slowly builds up to a quick-tempo climax marking an abrupt transition from order to disorder. Kurosawa's camera captures a line of feudal lords sitting almost at a right angle to it and then yet another line, to convince us of Washizu's powerful control of them, upon which his stability rests, but which is now in danger of weakening. Washizu slowly drinks his sake, and the camera cuts to the two empty seats. He lowers his sake cup with equal slowness, and then the camera takes in

Washizu and the empty seats to reassert his link with the murder of Miki and at the same time foreshadow his subsequent emotional faltering. The camera slowly tracks up toward Washizu, as if stalking his true feelings or waiting for him to crack.

Suddenly, Washizu sees Miki's ghost and staggers back. The appearance of the phantom externalizes Washizu's guilt and paves the way for the subsequent dramatization of the working of his mind. The camera follows Washizu's movement slowly, in ironic contrast to his inner emotional quaking, almost to the extent of aestheticizing his psychology. The empty seat and Washizu are recaptured yet again to emphasize his part in the murder of Miki.

Donald Richie mentions that Kurosawa's sparse use of close-ups in favor of long shots is influenced by the technique of *Noh* drama.[16] However, in this scene the camera moves right in and seems to explore Washizu's face; his features work to express horror and dismay, even as he tries to say, without undue emphasis, "I wonder what has become of Miki." The camera cuts to Asaji's face, which is a study in control: static, cold, and pretentious, like a *Noh* mask. There follows a crosscutting between Washizu's horrified face in close-up and the empty seat. We see Miki's ghost again from Washizu's perspective. This slow presentation of Washizu's inner tumult then suddenly breaks into rapid action. Washizu, feeling cornered, moves quickly across the hall, while the camera is stationary. Now the camera starts moving to take him fumbling with his sword. In contrast to the beautiful control of the old man's dancing shortly before, Washizu's movements suggest a madman's frantic gesticulations, a sort of dance macabre of suppressed guilt and horror.

The rest of the cinematic action centers around Washizu's alienation not only from his lords but also from his surroundings. All the guests have fled. The camera takes note of the empty tables. After Washizu's page leaves the hall, we are given an extreme long shot of the profile of Washizu facing his wife, which captures a sense of their alienation. An assassin arrives with Miki's head, and Lady Asaji leaves the room. Horrified by the news that Miki's son has escaped unharmed, Washizu kills the assassin. All of this occurs while Washizu is shown at one side of the screen. Now the camera backs off, centering him alone in the huge banquet hall. We see a center front long shot of Washizu standing between the two daises. Even more telling is the background wall of verticals broken by horizontal stripes; the visual composition is so balanced and stable that it enhances the protagonist's aberration and disorder. Thus, Washizu's second encounter with the two worlds of his destiny ends in an ironic view of static orderliness.

We are prepared for yet another encounter with the phantom world of prophecy and events ironically "squared." The raging wind merging with a murmur of servants' voices, the enemy's banners crackling angrily, lightning striking the castle, and Washizu's hysterical cry at the death of his newborn child—these acoustic elements presented in the prior scene are an ominous prelude to the final scene of phantasmagorical reality.

A thunderstorm heralds the second appearance of the witch. Lightning flickers in the forest. As the camera sweeps along the trees, sinister laughter merges with the thunder, and the witch with her white hair gleaming runs through the forest. In contrast to the previous phantasmagorical scene, here Washizu's moral chaos is exposed through movement set against a scene of natural disorder.

Instead of finding himself an equal to the witch, Washizu now finds himself a helpless victim whose fate is in her prophecy. Repeated intercutting between a medium shot of the witch laughing in the forest and a close-up or a medium shot of Washizu angry and frustrated expresses both Washizu's closeness to her and his wavering self-confidence. The witch prophesies that he will not be destroyed unless the forest marches on his castle.

Ghosts come out from different directions one after another, and Washizu struggles to get away from them. In his first encounter with the witch, it was Washizu who courageously fought his way out, shooting arrows into the lightning and urging his horse onward. In contrast, what we see now is circular motion as Washizu turns round and round to escape the encircling ghosts. The spatial limit of his movement and his disoriented turning effectively articulate a loss of control and his consequent entrapment in the wheel of fate. The circular movement later recurs as Washizu's enemy encircles his castle and again most dramatically as soldiers surround the staggering Washizu in the final scene. This can be taken as an archetypical pattern of the spinning wheel of fate. The trees filmed slightly askew, and the flashing lightning coming from different directions, also visualize Washizu's moral distortion.

We have observed in this scene that the phantasmagorical reality has two thematic functions; it not only expresses Washizu's entrammelment in moral chaos but also stresses the inevitability of his fate. At this stage we come to ponder whether Washizu's commitment to evil is internally or externally motivated. The film's action leads us to believe that Washizu's subjugation to evil is the result of his desire for power. But when we come to reflect on the recurrent circular motion and the images of the spinning wheel and the spider's web, the symbolic associations pose the existence of an uncontrollable fate as another perspective. Kurosawa leaves this problem to our judgment, because his primary concern is with the process of Washizu's moral decay not with the issue of the internalization or the externalization of his motive.

The rest of the film quickly leads us through a series of powerful dramatizations of Washizu's downfall. In contrast to the phantasmagorical scenes, in which his psychology is externalized, the last sequence focuses on more realistic, tangible visualization of moral chaos occasionally interspersed with supernatural elements. We see long shots of soldiers approaching and circling the castle. The circular movement, again suggestive of Washizu's entrapment in evil, dominates. As he holds a council of war with his generals, a flock of ravens fly into the audience room and circle through it. The castle itself becomes the chaotic center as though it were objectifying Washizu's own internal chaos. Lady Asaji's loss of the child and her consequent madness reveal sterility and confusion as forces at work in the castle. When the enemy attacks, the spears and the banners carried by Washizu's retainers are scattered everywhere, displaying his ineptitude in exercising leadership. His physical movement from the top of the castle down to the ground and his final dramatic demise as his throat is pierced by arrows combine with the enemy's circular movement to make his inevitable self-destruction particularly powerful.

The film ends the way it began: the choral incantation informs us again of the outcome of soaring ambition and the mutability of human affairs *(mujō)*. Then the screen presents the post stone of the castle. Just as the chorus at the end of the phantom *Noh* play prepares the audience for the shift from the supernatural to the tangible reality, here the chorus, aided by the visual image, helps us to emerge from the glimpse of the phantasmagorical world that the film has created for us.

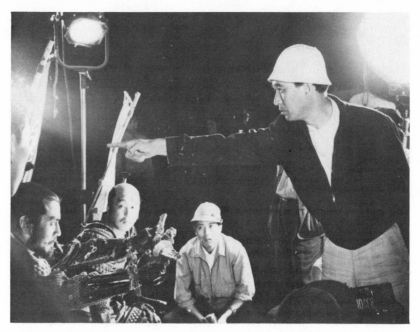

Throne of Blood (1957). Kurosawa directing the woodland scene.

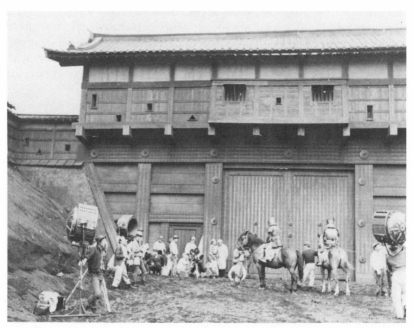

Throne of Blood (1957). The set of the castle gate built at the foot of Mt. Fuji.

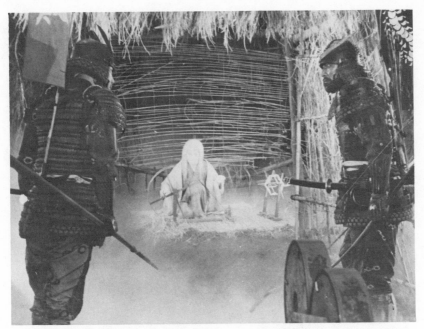

Throne of Blood (1957). Washizu (Toshirō Mifune), the witch (Chieko Naniwa), and Miki (Minoru Chiaki).

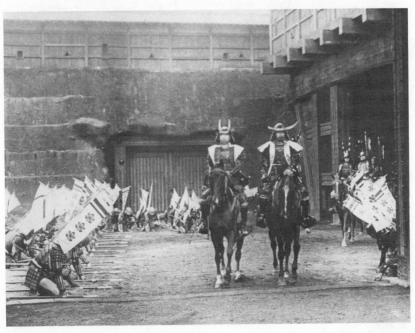

Throne of Blood (1957). Washizu (Toshirō Mifune) and Miki (Minoru Chiaki) after their victory.

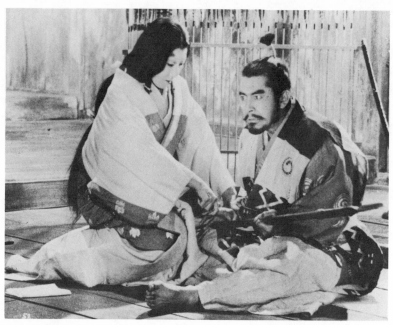

Throne of Blood (1957). Washizu (Toshirō Mifune) and Lady Washizu (Isuzu Yamada).

NOTES

1. J. Blumenthal, "Macbeth into *Throne of Blood, Sight and Sound* 34 (Autumn 1965):190–95.

2. Charles Bazerman, "Time in Play and Film: *Macbeth* and *Throne of Blood,*" *Literature/Film Quarterly* 5 (Fall 1977):339–45.

3. Marsha Kinder, *"Throne of Blood:* A Morality Dance," *Literature/Film Quality* 5 (Fall 1977): 339–45. Kinder points out three important visual polarities, which serve as an effective medium for transforming the dramatic action into "a kind of morality dance." The first polarity, she argues, involves action and observation between which the individual characters vacillate. The second polarity involves the palpable physical world based on "insubstantial light and shadow," and the third polarity is that of motion and stasis, that is, "the moving image within a static frame."

4. Roger Manvell, "Akira Kurosawa's *Macbeth, The Castle of the Spider's Web,*" *Shakespeare and the Film* (New York: Praeger, 1971), pp. 103–13. This essay is also devoted to the critical summary of both Blumenthal's criticism of the film and Satō's analysis of choreography derived from the *Noh* tradition. A more detailed treatment of Kurosawa's choreographic and spatial concern is found in Satō's *Kurosawa Akira no Sekai* [The World of Akira Kurosawa] (Tokyo: Saniichi Shobō, 1969), pp. 203–14.

5. Donald Richie, *The Films of Akira Kurosawa* (Berkeley: University of California Press, 1970), pp. 115–24. In addition to offering a key insight into these traditional elements of *Noh,* Richie analyzes Kurosawa's restrictive imagery and demonstrates how it is stylistically bolstered by his concise cinematography.

6. Satō, *Kurosawa Akira no Sekai* [The World of Akira Kurosawa], pp. 209–10.

7. In some cases, the protagonist cannot liberate himself from suffering because his attachment to this earth is too strong. One of the prime examples is found in *Motomezuka* [The Sought-for Tomb].

8. *Kurozuka* is a phantom *(mugen) Noh* play whose author is anonymous. In the first part of the play a party of traveling monks encounters an old woman who curses her fate of being born into the human world, as she spins the wheel. They ask for shelter overnight in her thatched hut. In the second part, the woman reveals her true identity in a demon form and engages the monks in combat, only to be defeated in the end.

9. In this case, it refers to a dance performed independently from the *Noh* play as entertainment for the banquet.

10. The opening passage reads:

"In the sound of the bell of the Gion Temple echoes the impermanence of all things. The pale hue of the flowers of the teak-tree show the truth that they who prosper must fall. The proud ones do not last long, but vanish like a spring-night's dream. And the mighty ones too will perish in the end, like dust before the wind."

Trans. by Donald Keene in *Japanese Literature* (New York: Grove Press, 1955), p. 78.

11. Satō, pp. 210–11. Roger Manvell also briefly refers to this aspect of the characters' facial pause mentioned by Satō. See *Shakespeare and the Film,* p. 105.

12. Kinder, *"Throne of Blood:* A Morality Dance," p. 342.

13. Richie, *The Films of Akira Kurosawa,* p. 120.

14. Ibid.

15. Ibid.

16. Ibid., pp. 117–21.

PART 5
TIME

9

Time, Sex, and Politics in Yoshida's *Eros plus Massacre*

Yoshishige Yoshida is considered a representative figure of the Japanese *nouvelle vague* movement. Ever since his debut with *Good for Nothing* [Rokudenashi, 1960], his creative activity has chiefly been directed toward various problems of "Eros" that are inherent in Japanese society. For example, his second and third films, *Dry Earth* [Chi wa Kawaite Iru, 1960] and *Bitter End of a Sweet Night* [Amai Yo no Hate, 1961], picture sexual manipulation as the epitome of contemporary society. In *Akitsu Spa* [Akitsu Onsen, 1964], Yoshida presents city life as detrimental to pure, healthy love, and his *Forbidden Love* [Mizu de Kakareta Monogatari, 1965] explores the dark aspects of the Japanese family system as manifested in an incestuous relationship. *Woman of the Lake* [Onna no Mizuumi, 1966] and *The Affair* [Jōen, 1967] intricately describe both the carnal and the platonic relationships of women. *Farewell to Summer Light* [Saraba Natsu no Hikari, 1968] and *Affair in the Snow* [Juhyō no Yoromeki, 1968] explore the inexplicable role of love in a woman's triangular relationship with her husband and lover.

Yoshida's two subsequent films, *Eros plus Massacre* [Erosu purasu Gyakusatsu, 1969] and *Heroic Purgatory* [Rengoku Eroika, 1970], mark a radical departure in his films in that they not only reveal a new direction in his treatment of "*Eros*"—its interaction with politics—but also introduce his experimentation with temporal and spatial concerns. Ōshima preceded Yoshida in exploring the theme of sex and revolution of sex and politics in such films as *Violence at High Noon* [Hakuchū no Tōrima, 1966], *Sing a Song of Sex* [Nihon Shunka-kō, 1967], and *Death by Hanging* [Kōshikei, 1968]. However, Yoshida's *Eros plus Massacre* rises above these works in terms of a Proust-like treatment of time.[1]

171

Concerning the complex conceptualization of time employed in *Eros plus Massacre*, Tadao Satō mentions *Ikiru* (1954) as a possible source of inspiration, citing Yoshida's own criticism of the Kurosawa film. Yoshida claims that the funeral of Watanabe in *Ikiru* is a kind of farce but that, because of the farcical element, we sense "the curve of severe action as if an object jumped out at us from the inside of this curve." However, according to Satō, Yoshida's criticism of *Ikiru* applies to his own work:

> Just as the last half of *Ikiru* is concentrated on the survivors' discussion of the deceased Watanabe, so *Eros plus Massacre* focuses on the contemporary persons who act, thinking of the dead—the anarchist Sakae Ōsugi, Noe Itō and others who lived in the Taishō era. While those who are dead represent a splendid way of living and dying, those who contemplate upon the past characters' action are aimless in their living, and are literally groping for their way in the dark. The common denominator in these two films, beyond the superficial similarity, is that they are very critical films in that the living criticize the dead, and vice versa.[2]

Satō's criticism is rewarding as it establishes time as a point of departure for examining Yoshida's contextual framework for *Eros plus Massacre*.

A further remark of Yoshida's is central to our understanding of the conceptual basis of his thematic treatment of time in the film:

> As Bergson said, our present may be exposed, floating on the clear surface of our hidden memory. However, this memory is never constant and fixed. If we leave the past as it is, it will remain vacant forever. We capture the present, working on the past, negating or reconstructing it, and we continue to live.
>
> The same thing can be said about our treatment of space. Don't we consider it to be free in movement and changeable instead of thinking of it as a mere expansion, and compulsively weave it into our daily lives?[3]

The action of *Eros plus Massacre* centers around two groups of people from different time periods: Sakae Ōsugi, an advocate of free love in the 1910s (Taishō period) and his three women (Yasuko, Noe, and Itsuko) on one hand, and Eiko and her two lovers (Unema and Wada) living in the 1960s on the other.[4] As Eiko becomes engrossed in her imaginary world, there occurs a dynamic interaction of the past (1916–23) and the present (1969). Furthermore, through her imagination, the past is continually revaluated, one imaginary version being replaced by another, and the reinforcement of the past and the present by each other becomes more complex. Significantly enough, Ōsugi and his women are not entirely the creation of Eiko's imagination, as Satō points out.[5] Hence, rather than acting the way Eiko imagines, they assert the autonomy of their own imaginations and start imagining their past experience, even transcending the temporal dimension altogether and putting themselves in the present. For example, Noe arrives in Tokyo, wearing an outfit of the Taishō period, riding a bullet train, a product of 1964. Then, she takes a ricksha in front of the modern Tokyo Station. Thus, the film frequently presents the framework of imagination within imagination.

This complex network of time is buttressed by Yoshida's adept use of crosscutting and space. The rapid crosscutting between the past and the present augments a sense of close interaction of the two distinctly different historical periods. Various technical elements make Yoshida's dramatization of time more substantial: the frequent, abrupt decentralization of characters, the contrast between black and white, and the traditional "staginess" as revealed in slow motion and vertical and horizontal lines in the props (such as *shōji* door and the wall). Thus, the continual mixing of contemporary and the Taishō periods makes this film one of the most "challenging" to be produced in the 1960s.

Furthermore, there is a constant vicillation in time within the Taishō period itself: we are shifted back and forth between 1916 (the fifth year of Taishō) and 1923 (the twelfth year of Taishō). Yoshida considers these two years to be what connects Ōsugi and Noe, as 1916 marked the beginning of their involvement with Eros and 1923 the time of their massacre.[6] This aspect of temporal dimension also contributes to the viewer's intellectual involvement.

Indeed, some critics have wondered aloud if Yoshida himself knew exactly what he was up to when he made this film. Others point to Yoshida's debt to *Dernière Année à Marienbad* and *L'Avventura*. My own view is that a careful study of the time framework in the film shows a degree of control and ingenuity all Yoshida's own. It offers the viewer more than a merging of two time periods separated by forty years; it offers a deft but difficult double merger. It is as if an earlier period had been recalled to examine its values (here, of Eros) in light of a later period which itself is gravely in doubt, and questions itself in the presence of a special "double-take" of time.

It has been argued that, like Kurosawa's *Rashomon*, *Eros plus Mas-*

sacre questions reality. However, in my view, the time framework
and levels of reality are used to explore another problem: "What
does Eros mean?" How is it related to politics?" By presenting both
Eiko's actual and imaginary worlds as the center of consciousness,
Yoshida offers two distinctly different equations: Eros = the basis
for political revolution, specifically, women's liberation; and
Eros = decadence and inertia. The barrenness of love in
contemporary society is the motif that Yoshida has persistently
kept pursuing in earlier films like *Akitsu Spa* (1964) and *Woman of the
Lake* (1966). In *Eros plus Massacre*, too, he explores the same motif
through a different method of presentation: heavy reliance on a new
treatment of time.

The first view of Eros is represented by the Taishō characters
brought back to life (and present history) through Eiko's imagination. The second view concerns the characters of the 1960s. Both
views are of course considerably modified by the startling autonomy of the imagination of the characters from the Taishō period,
just as we, the detached observers, discover that our sense of all
that is going on is considerably modified by our jumping in and out
(to borrow Yoshida's image) of these imaginary worlds.

Needless to say, imagination is not so systematic. As might be
expected, the film's progression is not so straightforwardly
schematic. A scene-by-scene study of the action reveals unexpected, and often quite difficult, tricks of insight—what we have
called "double-takes"—played by imagination on itself. Yoshida
has prepared a sequence that repays study.

Eros plus Massacre opens with the bustling roar of a busy section of
Fukuoka City. Yet this roar is interspersed with momentary si-
lences. In the juxtaposition of roar and silence Yoshida establishes
the universal character of contemporary society: death in life. Eiko
stops a young girl at a crowded intersection of a street and starts
questioning her. Eiko's voice rings out: "Are you Mako? You're a
daughter of Noe Itō, a mistress of the anarchist Ōsugi, who was
massacred with him in the confusion of the 1923 Great Earthquake?" Disregarding the young girl's bewildered face, Eiko continues to ask her questions.

When the young girl shakes her head, the setting quickly metamorphoses into what seems to be a large studio. We see the same
girl seated on a chair placed in the middle of the room. From Eiko's
subsequent interview, we come to learn more about Noe Itō, the
object of her imagination. We also realize that this young girl is a
link for Eiko as she tries to evaluate the past in terms of the present.

The interview reveals Noe as a dynamic figure in her day: "Noe Itō married three times during her life of twenty-eight years. After her marriage to the poet Jun Tsuji, her third husband, she became a lover of Sakae Ōsugi, leaving her husband and two children. She later became involved in the tragic incident at Hikagejaya Inn, in which another lover of Ōsugi's, Itsuko, stabbed him. She was also an active young contributor to *Seitō* [Bluestocking]. . . ."

Mako, who turns out to be the creation of Eiko's imagination but at the same time seems actually to exist, arouses our critical curiosity. During the interview, Yoshida presents only the young girl's face, shifting from right to left. This constant decentering of the girl has already established the ambiguous nature of Eiko's imagination, which is sustained throughout the film. When Eiko repeatedly asks the young girl whether she loves her mother, we encounter a prime example of Yoshida's use of cinematography in temporal transition. The camera quickly cuts from the girl to Eiko, who is suddenly illuminated by the light from the ceiling. Then, the screen becomes dim, and we are introduced to Eiko's recollection: the dark lobby of the Haneda Airport where a middle-aged director, Unema, is seeing her off on her flight to Fukuoka. She proceeds to the departure gate and disappears into the bright exterior symbolic of her search, linking past and present.

When Yoshida cuts back to the large studio, we, though unconvinced, begin to guess that the interview, and hence the young girl must be real and Noe's daughter, in spite of the impossible discrepancy in her age. Eiko persists in her attempt to reconstruct the past through the interview. When she suggests that Mako became unsteady when her parents left her, the camera's movement becomes uneasy, suggesting that Eiko is suddenly dizzy.

Now, in Eiko's imagination, time quickly shifts to the past: Noe is walking slowly along a beach covered with low pine trees. The white-caps and the wind blowing over the desert-like beach are soundless. The silence suggests the austerity of Eiko's imagination. Suddenly, the film moves back to the present and we see the young girl covering her face with her hands as the interview draws close to its end. For the first time, the young girl speaks. She denies that she is Mako and insists that she does not know who her mother is. As she slowly moves her hands, a glittering light comes through the spaces between her fingers until the screen is completely white. This makes a smooth transition to a mood appropriate for the exuberant yet fleeting passion that flared between the two lovers: Noe Itō and Sakae Ōsugi. Thereupon, the main title, *Eros plus Massacre*,

appears. An epigraph follows, expressing the director's intention
clearly:

> This film is about the conversation of contemporary youths; with
> degenerate pleasure they talk about the revolution and erotica involving
> Sakae Ōsugi . . . and Noe Itō. . . .

The epigraph also mentions "ambivalent participation" in the film's
action as our basic rhetorical stance. The term is rather puzzling,
but as the film itself suggests, a proper perspective needed for us is
a combination of intellectual involvement and emotional detachment. This is probably what Yoshida means by this term.

The setting moves ahead to March 3, 1969, in the Hotel Oriental
in Tokyo. In ironic contrast to the ceremonial elegance implied by
the doll festival on March 3, and to the prime vibrant love the
earlier epigraph implies, the screen shows us a spiritless sex act.
When Unema is making love to Eiko lying naked on a bed, her eyes
reveal a cold indifference to him. Meanwhile on a sofa nearby,
completely unconcerned, Wada is reading an English newspaper.
The paper is filled with various traumatic incidents around the
world—a counteroffensive by Arab guerrillas, stagnation of the
Paris conference on a cease-fire in Vietnam, and so on.

Wada's subsequent talk with Unema articulates contemporary
man's existence devoid of human love: empty time simply spreads
before him, and he cannot fill it in any way that would make his
existence significant. Wada himself sees time as simply an expanse
of vacuum. In response to Unema's remark that Wada is uncertain
of his future, Wada says that to him the future is simply an extension of his paralytic existence, as there is nothing he likes to do. In
Eiko's ensuing conversation with Unema, Yoshida explicitly describes her self-centered attitude: she claims that she does not love
anybody, that loving is insignificant. After sex, Eiko bathes. As she
embraces herself in the shower, Yoshida's camera, panning across
her body, suggests that self-love is the only love she knows.

By frequently presenting Eiko's vacant and Wada's cold eyes
during the sex scene, Yoshida has given us a sense of spiritual
vacuum, in which sex is a matter of "performance," a mechanical
routine expressive of contemporary standards. This dehumanized
sex is captured with vivid irony at the end of the scene when Wada,
still seated in his chair, burns the paper he has read. Following his
line of sight, the camera captures Unema and Eiko making love
behind the flame in another room with the door wide open. This

flame, an ironic symbol of sexual passion, contrasts with the lovelessness we see.

Eiko's imaginings now take a sort of fantasy escape from the indifferent lovemaking. We are in the world of Sakae Ōsugi and Noe Itō. The opening shot of cherry blossoms floating in the wind and a soft background of piano music establish the lyrical mood appropriate for their romantic love in striking contrast to the cold contemporary love just presented. Associated with perishability, the traditional Japanese image of cherry blossoms emphasizes the nature of this kind of love: so alive that it is doomed to destruction. For example, when Noe mentions that Ōsugi's eyes reflect the cherry blossoms, we are reminded of Eiko and Wada's lifeless eyes in the earlier scene. Moreover, in terms of the director's exploration of time, this image brings these lovers the memories of their own past and thus leads them into a recaptured time frame quite independent of Eiko's imagination. The cherry blossoms thus serve as a prelude to the complex temporal framework of imagination within imagination.

After the opening shot we see Ōsugi and Noe coming out of a grove in Hibiya Park where the cherry blossoms are in full bloom. As Noël Burch also points out, the blossoms dominate the screen while only the heads of the two occupy the lower portion of the screen.[7] This decentralizing of the lovers pervasively reminds us of the dramatic nature of their love symbolized by the blossoms. Ōsugi stops and looks at them. They take him back to his past: the spring of three years ago. On 24 January 1913, his revolutionary comrades, Shūsui Kōtoku and eleven others, were hanged for treason, while Ōsugi and two other comrades, who were in prison at that time, were spared. Even in the middle of that spring, he remembers, the cherry blossoms did not bloom, as if in sympathy for his comrades' death. Ōsugi is now an anarchist whose every moment is watched by government spies.

The subsequent conversation between Ōsugi and Noe tells us what has brought her so close to him. Noe, who was involved in the revolutionary magazine, *Seitō* [Bluestocking], which often explored such social issues as land reform, had written to him for advice. As soon as Noe utters the words, "My cherry blossoms," the scene switches to a world of Noe's fantasy, again, independent of Eiko's imagination. We see Noe then, an eighteen-year-old girl, coming along the corridor of the Shinbashi Station. She has just arrived in the metropolis from the countryside on a modern bullet train; she wears a plain kimono with her hair in a braid, the appearance common among girls in the 1910s. The brief projection of the Taishō figure against the contemporary setting reminds us of the past and the present.

As her subsequent talk with Ōsugi reveals, she escaped from her home prior to her wedding because she did not want to bind herself to the social conventions of her village as a housewife. In her recollection, she is on her way to Tsuji, her former schoolteacher, who will marry her. When she comes out of the station and mounts a *ricksha*, cherry blossoms in full bloom come into her sight. They externalize the hope and joy with which she regards her new life in Tokyo, and at the same time they foreshadow the fleeting nature of her liberation. Her recollection continues, and we learn that Noe took over the journal *Seitō* when the editor Akiko Hiraga decided to resign. Still in her recollection, Noe is introduced by Akiko to Itsuko Masaoka, Ōsugi's mistress. Inside the house that serves as the editorial office of the journal the three women talk. Yoshida's camera captures the low ceiling and effectively transmits a sense of claustrophobia signifying the oppression they experience and fight against through the journal.

Noe opens the window. Peonies, plum, and bamboo in the snow-covered garden strike her eyes. Yoshida's presentation of Noe's world is radically different from that of Eiko's world. While Noe is portrayed in the context of natural phenomena, symbolic of her affinity for nature, Eiko is always presented against the gloomy fabricated setting characteristic of her insipid world. This contrast significantly reflects their attitudes toward sex: Noe's freedom and vitality counterpoised with Eiko's sense of ennui and stultification.

Yoshida quickly moves us from Noe's memory to the contemporary setting. In Unema's studio, Eiko and Wada are idly watching each other while Unema is busily directing a film. This scene demonstrates Yoshida's effective use of imagery of light to project death associated with contemporary love. For example, Unema works in a strong white light suggestive of the barren world of contemporary man. When his camera begins to move, its mechanical eye symbolizes the paranoia of contemporary man. Yoshida's subsequent presentation of Eiko's dizziness in the light coming from the studio reinforces this symbolic implication.

Later in this scene the light image is presented in another form. Wada lights a match. Eiko says that playing with fire is his means of escape from direct confrontation with adulthood. The fire image again represents wish fulfillment—sexual passion, of which contemporary man has become incapable. Thus, when Eiko sexually challenges Wada saying, "Can you burn me? You're going to burn me," his response is only silence. The pervasive sense of the mechanization of sex is further augmented by the wire dolls, which are the actors in Unema's film. Irony ends this scene when he orders a doll to smile, shouting that it can smile better than a human actor.

This mechanization of sex enters another phase when Hinoshiro, a detective, comes into the studio to tell Eiko that she is a prime suspect in a recent prostitution case. Eiko laughs cynically while on the sound track we hear Unema shout at the doll: "Laugh! You can laugh better than a human being." Here Yoshida's use of contrast is evident. In 1969, Eiko, in her early twenties, commits herself to free love, not for reasons of real fulfillment, but only out of boredom. Sex is figuratively "prostituted." Concomitantly, in 1916 Noe, in her early twenties, left her husband to be with Ōsugi for a genuine enrichment of her life. The ensuing shot presents the sparkling light and a cloudlike smoke caused by a box of matches Wada has lit. His mechanical voice expresses the boredom of living: "I don't have anything to do, though it does not matter."

The action now shifts to one day in February 1916, a month before the meeting between Ōsugi and Noe at Hibiya Park earlier presented. Yoshida's filmic transition is full of contrast. A wooden Japanese house has replaced the modern studio, and elegant flute music has succeeded the metalic sound of Unema's rolling camera. Tsuji, Noe's husband, is playing a flute, sitting on the veranda. Its plaintive tune vibrates through the cold February air, expressing Tsuji's solitude and preparing us for Yoshida's subsequent exploration of conjugal discord between Tsuji and Noe.

The following dialogue between them, aided by Yoshida's cross-cutting, discloses their variant views on freedom of women and free love. Noe, now the established editor of *Seitō*, is ready to leave the house to work for the forthcoming issue. Noe says that Tsuji has not helped her with her journal. He answers that he has already given her all the help she needed, adding that all that he wants now is to stay away from her. While their conversation goes on, Yoshida's camera presents both Tsuji on the veranda and Noe within the frame of the center glass pane of the *shōji* door. This filmic composition clearly visualizes a distinct separation of values. Tsuji continues to condemn Noe's idea of women's liberation:

'Each time you open your mouth, you talk about women's liberation. Of course, their position must be improved. However, these days I

wonder if we have kept playing only with the slogan. Women's liberation, modern age, ego. . . . What do they mean? You, an advocate of
women's liberation, don't know how to run the house or raise our
children. . . . I certainly admire your ability to act. . . .

Noe contends that her husband himself has taught her Stillnell's
idea that one must not seek freedom in self-denial. When she is
talking, the camera stays on her face, while Tsuji is out of focus.
This take again reinforces their marital disharmony.

When the scene cuts back to the contemporary setting, we see
the staircase of a cheap hotel against a gloomy dirty wall. Eiko and
Hinoshiro, the middle-aged detective, climb the stairs and enter a
sparsely decorated room. The subsequent scene explores the issue
revolving around the central problem—the degeneration of sex
found in contemporary man. Eiko proceeds to reconstruct her
crime of prostitution. While Hinoshira's voice echoes tinnily on the
sound track, saying that she stripped off her clothes, Eiko takes off
her clothing piece by piece, as if she were enjoying it. While the
detective says, "You showed your merchandise," she starts moving
around the bed like a fashion model, demeaning her customer, who
is now seen lying there.

Since the reconstruction of the crime takes place in semidark-
ness, we see only the silhouette of her body. Reality and fantasy
now seem to interact. As the light emphasizes the skinny body of
the moving girl, we begin to wonder whether the girl we thought
was Eiko really is Eiko. We continue to be uncertain even as the
"crime" is reenacted. Hinoshiro's voice asks her how much she
charged her customer. Eiko answers that she has become tired of
this game. When his voice asks her name, we, for the first time,
understand the implication of the optical confusion which Yoshida
has deliberately created for us: contemporary people have lost their
identities. Eiko remarks: "It does not matter whether girl was me or
not. I don't care because I simply do not exist for me."

Having thus presented the sterility of love and the concomitant
loss of selfhood in the contemporary world. Yoshida quickly moves
back to the past. From this point on, the convergence of politics and
Eros becomes increasingly predominant. It is a winter day in the
so-called Winter Period of Socialism (from the end of the Meiji
period to the beginning of the Taishō period, i.e., the 1910s). We
see Ōsugi serving a term in prison. The opening shot of this scene
presents another prime example of Yoshida's spatial consideration
made effective by the alignment of black and white. Both sides of

the wall are stone walls; the one separated by iron bars and the other, dimly white, leading into darkness. The surrealistic atmosphere evoked by this alignment leads us to believe that the director is now presenting Ōsugi's recollection within Eiko's world of imagination.

Leaning against the iron bars, Ōsugi is arguing with his two fellow inmates. When Sakai, one of them, remarks that Ōsugi seems to emphasize the philosophy of *vita* but that he may be advocating the philosophy of sex, we vaguely sense Ōugi's equation of political freedom with sexual freedom. This sense of ours will be confirmed later in the film.

With ambivalent feelings about Ōsugi's political commitment, we are again shifted back to the contemporary period. Eiko and Wada are doing the bunny hop to some jazzy music against the background of what appears to be the foundation of a new building. Yoshida's cinematic concern manifests itself in shot sizes, architecture, and motion. The foundation is accentuated by both vertical and horizontal stripes. An extreme long shot of Wada against this desolate background again evokes the spiritual vacuum in which contemporary man finds himself. Wada says: "I have seen you making love to other men, but I've never slept with you myself." Eiko drily answers: "You're psychologically impotent." Wada denies it. They engage in erotic wordplay as a substitute for the real thing.

The progress of their imaginary-sex game in conveyed through images of the eyes. Eiko is presented as being afraid of looking into Wada's eyes, as if paranoia were another deterrent to love. Interestingly enough, when Wada, still in imagination, embraces her, their movement becomes a slow dance as if to remind us that we are still watching their world of fantasy.

The constant impingement of external events upon individual lives is also the deterrent to love in the ensuing scene. Wada, all of a sudden, discontinues the game. He tells Eiko that a crowd of people are running toward them. She looks around, but she cannot see anything in front of her except an empty field. Now their imagination takes another turn. They pretend that they have barely escaped from the crowd watching a serious accident caused by the sudden fall of a huge crane. Wada pretends to be a reporter and interviews Eiko, a "witness" to the accident. Wada's reporting is graphic. Holding an imaginary microphone in his hand, he describes "the ocean of blood and pieces of flesh, in addition to a small handbag containing a doll, an old victim's gift to her grandchild

lying in a ditch." We understand that this brutality is to be seen as
the condition of contemporary society, a state of callous indifference to traumatic events—a condition inimical to humane values.

The final scene of this section signifies the lifelessness of modern
love. Eiko starts running toward the empty field. Throwing the
microphone to the ground, Wada pursues her. The camera then
shifts to take Eiko and Wada lying on the ground, forming a cross.
A long shot of a real cross then moves from the center to the left of
the screen and yields to a medium shot of it in the center position.
These shots of the cross impress upon our minds the idea that the
death of love is a consequence of contemporary values.

The setting shifts again back to the Taishō period. It is an evening in March. Ōsugi is standing against an arch-shaped window,
facing Itsuko, one of his mistresses. They are in her boardinghouse,
a Western-style brick building constructed in the Meiji era. Again,
Yoshida's camera emphasizes the low ceiling, to which the windows almost reach. The imposing and almost claustrophobic atmosphere thus created foreshadows not only the ensuing tension
between Ōsugi and Itsuko but also the nature of their love, which is
doomed to destruction.

Their subsequent conversation explores the quadrangular relationship between Ōsugi, Itsuko, Noe and Yasuko. It also reveals
Ōsugi's and Itsuko's choices of action evolving around the central
problem of the film. Ōsugi frankly admits that he loves both Itsuko
and Noe as well as his wife, Yasuko. He claims that the three of
them can get along very well as long as they observe three conditions: "First, the three of you have to be economically independent.
Second, you have to let me live separately from you instead of
living with any one of you. Third, you must respect each other's
freedom, including that of sex."

Now it is clear that Ōsugi's solution to the central problem is the
association of freedom with free love, a revolutionary idea in
Taishō society. As the film's subsequent action shows, Itsuko's
solution is essentially similar to Ōsugi's. However, she proposes
three conditions that Ōsugi must observe in their pursuit of sexual
freedom. Challenging his desire to be open about their relationship
with his other mistresses and his colleagues, Itsuko persuades him
to keep it as secret as possible. We become aware that this condition
stems from a fear of openly flaunting social conventions. Her second condition is to avoid any onus of responsibility, especially
pregnancy. Ōsugi's orientation to sex, then, is complete freedom,
whil Itsuko's is attenuated freedom constrained within social
mores.

Silence is Itsuko's only answer to Ōsugi's question about her third condition. Again Yoshida relies heavily upon contrast for a temporal shift. This silence yields to the dialing of a telephone in a contemporary setting: the hustle and bustle of a coffee shop. We now see Eiko talking to Hinoshiro, the detective, who earlier questioned her. As Eiko tells him that she has acted as an intermediary for prostitution, Yoshida presents an extreme long shot of the two; they are decentered again. This device stresses their basic discord with their environment. Hinoshiro analyzes Eiko's agony in living. In a monotonous voice he tells her that she escapes into imagination to avoid the agony of her pointless existence. He is in effect saying that contemporary man can rebel only in imagination. Eiko still insists that there are two Eikos in her: an imaginary one, who acted as procurer for prostitution; and a real one, who is now talking to Hinoshiro. He tells her that he has already arrested the call-girl ring he was looking for, and advises her that she should stop indulging her imagination.

Still in the same time setting, the action shifts to a small apartment. It turns out to belong to Megumi, who has earlier contacted Eiko to tell her that she is about to commit suicide. Unema, whom Eiko has asked to see Megumi, is now facing her. Again we see the dynamic interaction of reality and imagination as Megumi exhibits a loss of all sense of time. She recalls to Unema what she has done since she got up at 6:37. Her full confession, which she makes in tears, articulates a fear of living aimlessly, deprived of human love.

After pausing on a bowl of fruit and round flowers, the symbols of life, the camera shifts to Megumi sobbing. The vertical lines of the room, which the camera has emphasized throughout the scene, externalize her sense of paranoia.[8]

Yoshida again takes us back to the Taishō period (April 1916). We see Tsuji's house where he is shown with his sister-in-law, Chiyoko, during Noe's absence. He takes out his flute and starts playing. Along Chiyoko's line of sight, the camera captures his solitude reinforced by the mournful music of a flute. Chiyoko closes the white *shōji* door and they make love to the sound of a train rattling by. Noe comes back. The camera captures her standing alone in the corridor outside the room. It is stationary on her, expressing the tension caused by her awareness of what is happening inside. She puts her hand on a pane of the *shōji* door. All of a sudden the scene shifts to the exterior to give us a shock: we see Noe swinging in a swing in the yard. The swing, a modern Western plaything, out of place in the traditional Japanese garden, indi-

cates the fusion of the contemporary and the Taishō periods, again
reminding us that we are still inside Eiko's world of imagination.
Inside the house Chiyoko is crying. Tsuji joins Noe in the garden.

The next two sections, still in Eiko's imagination, further explore
Noe's response to the central problem of the film. We learn that as a
result of her discovery of Tsuji's infidelity, she has now realized
that her free love can be achieved only through the breakdown of
her marriage. Noe's solitude and helplessness are effectively conveyed in a series of shots: Noe walking in the rain; Noe sobbing;
Noe pensive by the hedge of Ōsugi's house.

Noe's awakening is furthered when she and Yasuko face each
other in the small alley outside Ōsugi's house. They are shown
walking toward the camera, then standing in a puddle. Yasuko puts
it in plain words, contrasting women in general in the Taishō society with the woman Noe is trying to become: "You may have
changed the old *zōri* (straw sandals) for a new pair, but now your
feet are already muddy. . . . Look, you and I are in the muddy
pool."

The following section presents Noe's recollection within Eiko's
imagination, unfolding her open clash with Itsuko. We see Noe,
Ōsugi, and Itsuko in what appears to be a high-class boardinghouse. Noe has come here to tell Ōsugi that she is going to part
with him in order to become independent. Here, through Itsuko's
mouth, Yoshida articulates a radical idea of women's liberation
associated with the exploitation of sex. Itsuko demonstrates her
legitimate claim to monopolize Ōsugi's love since she has an earning
capacity as a journalist and takes care of both the destitute Ōsugi
and his wife.

But, ironically, the wall against which she is now leaning and the
low ceiling which Yoshida's camera has kept emphasizing, visualize
the limit of her revolt through sex against conventional Taishō
society. On the other hand, Ōsugi has silently been watching the
two women clash. He is unable to assert his claim, made earlier,
that sexual freedom is tantamount to political revolution. At this
stage, his idea of sexual freedom strikes us a mere expedient to
satisfy his lust.

When the location shifts, we see Noe walking on a street on the
same day in Eiko's world of imagination. All of a sudden, Noe sees
Ōsugi surrounded by his opponents and attacked with a stick. The
white monochrome, which suddenly dominates the screen, shocks
us, as though together with Noe we were experiencing each blow
that Ōsugi is suffering. At the same time, however, the abrupt

intrusion of the monochrome tells us that we are witnessing the action in Noe's imagination within Eiko's imagination. Ōsugi tries to reach for Noe but in vain. She herself falls to the ground. Our sense of the destruction of their love, thus awakened, is sustained until the later scene wherein Noe stabs Ōsugi, giving the final blow to their relationship.

Yoshida now brings us back to the contemporary setting. Eiko and Wada are again in Unema's studio. Throughout this section we see the recurrent fire image, this time the flame from the lighter, which burns bluntly in Wada's hand like a small weapon. When he confesses that he watched his mother's lover through the glass window of a bank in his childhood, we sense his distrust of her, which may have molded his distrust of women in his adulthood. Eiko snatches the lighter from his hand and starts burning the rolls of film hanging in the studio, one by one. They are safety film, however, and she only creates smoke. The symbolic implication of Eiko's gesture is clear: her inability to consummate her love with any man. Against her is the picture of two naked children kissing each other, which ironically pinpoints the modern adults' stultification of love. All of a sudden, darkness prevails. Eiko nonchalantly switches on a projector, and thereupon various scenes of the great Kanto Earthquake are projected on the screen.

Throughout the film Yoshida tries to convince us that we are watching the world of imagination displayed in Eiko's mind, that the past and the present work on each other like two electric currents attached to each other. One of Yoshida's methods of reinforcing this concept is to let the concrete image link the two. Thus, the films of the earthquake (1923), which Eiko has projected, take us back to the Taishō period. Next, when Wada starts reading aloud from a book on Ōsugi and Noe, which is in Eiko's possession, Yoshida presents another rapid succession of pictures of the earthquake. Wada's reading on the sound track and the montage on the screen combine to convey a sense of Eiko's close involvement with the Taishō figures. Wada reads:

> I saw, through the hedge in the backyard, Ōsugi and Noe going out together. Mako, who happened to be in my place, hurried out as soon as she saw them, but she returned very soon and said, 'My parents have gone out.' I never saw Ōsugi afterwards.

We have not been told who wrote this book, nor do we know what Eiko's link with the past will lead to. Our curiosity thus

aroused, we are again shifted back to the Taishō period and are
exposed to a more dynamic interaction of the past and the present.
Here, Eiko's imagination becomes more active. She fantasizes the
scene of Ōsugi's and Noe's murder, which actually took place on
the 16 September 1923.[9] First, we see Noe and Ōsugi sitting on the
chairs in a room, which seems to be a cell at the secret military
police headquarters. There follows a close-up of Noe and then one
of Ōsugi.

In order to make us aware that we are seeing through Eiko's
imagination, Yoshida again evokes the surreal atmosphere through
the alignment of black and white. First, Ōsugi's face is covered by a
pair of white gloved hands, effectively symbolizing death. He puts
the hands away only to be strangled by them. Next, Noe is
strangled by white-gloved hands, and Ōsugi is again strangled by
the same hands. Their faces rotate, as if to show the agony of
execution. After another shot of Noe being strangled by these
hands, there is a blackout, which evokes the sinister atmosphere
relevant to the execution. This yields to a shot of a boy (Sōichi
Tachibana, who was executed with Ōsugi and Noe) strangled by
the white-gloved hands. Repetition now becomes a dominant technique. There is one more presentation of Ōsugi and Noe being
strangled. Another blackout follows, emphasizing the termination
of the execution. Next, in the same surrealistic atmosphere, we see
Ōsugi and Noe attired in black against a white background. Again,
to emphasize Eiko's imagination, the filmic texture then completely
reverses itself. We now see Ōsugi's and Noe's white faces emerging
from the completely black background like *Noh* masks. Noe is trying to reach out for Ōsugi as if she were affirming her tie with him
at this last moment. Then, the filmic texture again changes, and we
see them now dressed in black against white.

Quickly thrust back to the studio in the present day, we find
Wada still reading the book against the black background. This
rapid transition convinces us that we have glimpsed Eiko's recreation of the execution of Ōsugi and Noe by the military police.
Wada's voice explains:

> The following day and the day after that, Mako came to see us. One
> day when she was here, a journalist came and took a picture of her.
> Then on the subsequent day the cruel death of Ōsugi was made
> public. . . . Whenever Mako saw one of us, she would say: "Father and
> mother died. My uncle and grandfather went to see them, and they are
> coming back by car today. . . ."

Wada closes the book. We know for the first time the title and the author as he reads them aloud: "Roan Uchida. *People I remember: The Last Moments of Ōsugi.* . . ." Through Wada's mouth Yoshida then questions Eiko's motive in becoming so involved with the Taishō figures: "What did you try to find in the dark stacks of the library? The past? The history of the record? . . ." Eiko does not answer. Yoshida's fine photography shows her against the white background, inviting an answer to Wada's question, and then this section abruptly ends with a blackout.

Still in a critical maze in our attempt to come up with a logical answer to Wada's question, we now witness an even more dynamic visual interaction of the past and the present. Against the hustle and bustle of Shinjuku, Eiko is interviewing Noe. Eiko starts by saying that she has been looking for Noe for a long time, that she has been to places as remote as Hakata to look for her. Eiko continues to say: "Do you understand what will happen to you tomorrow?" Thereupon, Noe answers: "Yes, now I can tell you what I will do tomorrow." Eiko says: "If you had not pursued Ōsugi further or if Itsuko Masaoka had won his love, do you think that you would have avoided death in the Great Earthquake of 1923?" Noe responds that she cannot change her life since what happened happened thanks to her way of living. We can now surmise that Eiko's goal is to reconstruct the past and thereby to give some meaning to the present and draw these two temporal points together as a continuum in the flux of time. We, however, in dismay, are unable to make sense of what is happening before our eyes.

Yoshida gives his own interpretation of this section as follows:

> Noe Itō was executed in 1923. Eiko is now living in 1969. However, did the lapse of these forty-six years really exist in Japan? Did these years really pass? What about history? This lapse of time is what a history book describes. The year 1923 and the year 1969—do these years and their worlds exist as separate physical entities? It seems accurate to say that the answer is no. Therefore, this section is not the world of Eiko's fantasy or the world of her imagination. It is the real world created through fiction.[10]

The last sentence is troubling, but Yoshida seems to negate our ordinary conception of time as a lineal progression. Instead, he seems to encourage us to conceive of time as a whirlpool, in which the past and the present are inextricably merged.

Eiko poses the last question: "What do you think of the last forty years?" The screen suddenly turns dark, as if to suggest what is happening to Noe's mind confronted with this question. As the flute music sounds again, a man and a child appear on the screen; they are Noe's husband and her son. As they cross a field of tall, white pampas grass, an extreme long shot of the two against the desolate atmosphere transmits a sense of their solitude after Noe's desertion. She tries to follow them as the flute music becomes louder. Father and son cross the screen, as Noe looks down at them near a cross. What crosses her mind is clear: remorse over her attempt to achieve sexual liberation by sacrificing them. She has carried a burden of guilt for the last forty-six years. After a shot of Noe leaning against the cross, the scene quickly shifts back to the Taishō period.

It is now early October in 1916 (the fifth year of Taishō). Ōsugi is facing his friend Kitamura in a hotel where he is now living with Noe. Kitamura has come here with one purpose: to advise Ōsugi as a friend and revolutionary colleague, that he should return to his wife. Ōsugi's vociferous self-defense expresses his response to the film's central problem:

> . . . what did revolution mean to us? It was a means by which we attempted to reach freedom. Our primary objective was to exterminate exploitation. But what does the private property system mean? It is the system which regards male/female relationship as absolute in the name of morality or rather, the system which regards property as basically hereditary. The problem lies in our determination to support this system. But to me, revolution means the complete destruction of this system. We are really becoming more distant from a revolution as long as we recognize, as sancrosanct, marriage, the family system, which is based upon matrimony, and the nation formed as a collective entity of families.

As Kitamura is ready to leave, failing in his mission, we see a long shot of Ōsugi at the furthest end of the corridor flanked by two walls. This composition makes us aware of his alienation from all his colleagues. His alienation from his wife is now verbally expressed, when he tells Kitamura to take care of her.

The scene shifts to Chigasaki Beach, where Aichō, the founder of *Seitō* (whom Noe replaced), her husband, and their child are walking. An extreme long shot of the three against the quiet, glittering waves of the ocean conveys the congenial harmony existing among them. After her brief encounter with Noe, we hear the flute music once again. Tsuji and his son walk across the screen from one end while Aichō's husband with a buggy walks across from the other. They meet in the center. This composition contrasts the former's solitude and the latter's happiness in marriage. It is precisely Noe's attempt that caused the destruction of her marriage and it is also Aichō's denial of her further attempt at women's liberation which brought about her matrimonial harmony.

The following several sections—Itsuko's sudden visit to the teahouse, Hikagejaya,[11] her reverie, and Noe's departure from the teahouse—are done through continuous crosscutting between the exterior and the interior. They reveal the intricate triangular affair of Ōsugi, Itsuko, and Noe. The clash of the three significantly leads us to realize the impossibility of combining Eros and politics, given Taishō social conventions. Here we also come again to doubt Ōsugi's motivation: though he claims that sexual liberation is a genuine force for political revolution, his own conduct thus far suggests a strong element of self-indulgence.

The film's action finally moves us to the climax, unfolding three versions of how Ōsugi is stabbed at Hikagejaya. Eiko's imagination reconstructs the first version, being faithful to the actual historical incident, in which Ōsugi was stabbed by one of his mistresses. At the beginning of this section we see Itsuko take a knife out and look at it. The serenity and quietude we have momentarily glimpsed in her earlier fantasy (of walking along a quay) lapse into turmoil when she starts stabbing Ōsugi in the neck. Next, we are again given Yoshida's dynamic camera movement appropriate to their physical struggle.

As blood streams out of his neck, she stabs her own throat with the same knife. They rotate round a pillar in the room. The camera's movement becomes uneasy as she staggers around the *shōji* door of their room and goes out to the corridor. Ōsugi and Itsuko combat in the corridor and then Ōsugi staggers along it, chasing after Itsuko. One by one *shōji* doors fall down while he keeps staggering, giving the impression of his roaming from one room to another in the teahouse.

The labyrinthine maze of love in which Ōsugi has entrapped himself by pursuing free love is obviously suggested, since Yoshida captures him lying among the fallen *shōji* doors as the camera rotates ninety degrees and rapidly. At the same time, we are rather surprised by the conventional outcome of Ōsugi's pursuit of Eros with Itsuko—his mistress's attempt to kill him. We now recall her earlier remark to Noe that Ōsugi was a part of her and that they possessed each other. This recollection, in turn, makes us aware that Itsuko's

homicidal attempt to monopolize his love is indicative of her conventional view of man/woman relationships, a far cry from radical
visions of free love.

Suddenly, the scene shifts back to the modern setting. It is
strongly accentuated by jazz on the sound track. Eiko and Wada are
still in Unema's studio. While their conversation goes on, Wada is
taking pictures of Eiko. We listen to his seemingly thematically
irrelevant monologue about the lover his mother had in the past.
We envision the correlation between the past and the present and
try to find a certain linkage between these young persons on one
hand and Ōsugi and his lovers on the other. When Wada says that
he is not interested in the past at all, that there is nothing for him to
do, he again expresses ennui as the sole predicament of his life.
After describing the homosexual tendencies of his mother's lover,
he suddenly explains that he now understands why this lover chose
death. He continues to say: "Then, he thought of death as the
greatest pleasure. Death reverses value." The death image is now
visually presented as Wada plays with a noose and pretends to hang
himself. Eiko's voice echoes: "What reverses the value?" It implies
her preoccupation with death, specifically with Ōsugi's tragic death
in his pursuit of free love.

Thus, convinced of the continuity of the past and the present, we
are taken to the second version of how Ōsugi was stabbed at the
teahouse. This version is also Eiko's creation and tells us "how
Ōsugi would have interpreted the actual historical incident at the
teahouse."[12] Eiko tries to interpret his fatal injury with her imagination highly influenced by Wada's earlier remark on death as su-
preme pleasure.

In contrast to the quick, unfaltering movement of Ōsugi and
Itsuko we witnessed in the first version, a quiet, slow movement,
interspersed with a fierce physical struggle, dominates in this version. The low-angled camera shows Ōsugi sleeping with his head
toward the lower edge of the screen. Itsuko, who sits near him,
quietly takes a dagger out from its sheath. In an almost balletlike
stylistic fusion of the static and the mobile, Yoshida's camera articulates the outcome of Ōsugi's relationship with Itsuko. Ōsugi
opens his eyes and asks her if she has to kill him. She replies that
there is no other choice. She quietly approaches him on her knees
and points the dagger at his chest. It looks like a white sword of
justice.

Their ensuing conversation reveals their views on death. Itsuko
considers death to be the inevitable outcome of their quadrangular

love. On the other hand, Ōsugi defends his idea of death as the ultimate form of ecstasy as well as his philosophical equation of revolution with self-denial. After his defense, the white *shōji* doors appear behind them again. This time, instead of closing upon the lovers, they are stationary. Their stillness and whiteness correspond to the solemnity and serenity which Ōsugi considers to be an integral part of death.

Next we see the rhythmic variation provided by the characters' gestures; the static movement of the two abruptly turns into dynamic action, then again into static. Ōsugi and Itsuko struggle in the corridor again, and then, as if we were caught in an optical illusion, we see them in a bathhouse. In his reverie Ōsugi confesses his part in a knife fight, in which he caused himself to be stabbed by a juvenile delinquent. He says: "I fell when he attacked me." Itsuko responds: "You knew exactly what would become of you." The camera is slightly askew, making us uneasy. We detect a correlation between what happened to Ōsugi in the past knife fight and what will happen to him now. We see him in the bathtub, and the camera pans down upon him. His stomach is stabbed. His recollection, "My entire body got cold suddenly," parallels what is happening to him now.

We are again back in the modern setting—Unema's studio with modern music on the sound track. This time, too, Yoshida shows Wada taking pictures of Eiko, reinforcing the sense of paranoia as the plight of lovers. The fire image, an ironic index of the barrenness of love, is reintroduced both verbally and visually. Eiko, offering Wada a lighter, says: "Can you set fire to me?" She takes off her clothes, and Wada takes pictures of her nude body lying on the floor. Eiko's repetitive remark, "You can't set fire, can you?" continues, as if she were trying to arouse his passion for her.

Yoshida has persistently emphasized the motif of the film—the sterility of love in contemporary society. Thus, Eros here is warped into a means of a woman's exploitation of man—a sexual game, which is itself the only stimulant that works for the sexually exhausted/ depressed men. Eiko snatches the lighter from Wada and sets fire to her nylon stockings. Next, we see Wada embrace and kiss her as the flame spreads over the white wall behind them. They fall together, and the flame becomes stronger, ironically signifying the sexual gratification that they have tried in vain to attain.

Yoshida then moves us back to the Taishō era and the third version of the way Ōsugi was stabbed. According to Satō, this is Yoshida's own version of the Hikagejaya incident projected into

Eiko's imagination.[13] Here we have Osugi with both of his lovers—
Noe and Itsuko. Significantly, the two women's views of free love,
which they consider an important step toward women's liberation,
are at stake. Exposing themselves to their impulse and jealousy, the
two reveal the inappropriateness of their initial choices of action in
relation to the central problem. Unlike rational women's liberation-
ists, Itsuko and Noe stage a knock-down, drag-out battle over their
man.

The opening shot presents Itsuko lifting a dagger with her shaking hand and trying to stab Ōsugi. To our surprise, Ōsugi is still
alive, with his eyes wide open. At this moment, the *shōji* door is
abruptly opened, and there stands Noe. Yoshida's camera first
shows the inflamed hatred and enmity with which Noe and Itsuko
stare at each other. Then it focuses on Itsuko looking at the dagger
in her hand as it reflects the white light from the window. It glitters
as if it were ready to absorb Ōsugi's life.

Yoshida then presents Itsuko trying fervently to stab Ōsugi only
to find her hand shaking. She goes to the window, through which
light is streaming in. It is not only a break in tension but also a
revelation to us. The light seems to signify Itsuko's tragic realization of the futility of her quest of free love. The dagger now drops
from her hand to become a mere metal fragment shining bluntly on
the floor. Noe comes closer and closer to her and explains why she
did not stab Ōsugi.

We now proceed to Itsuko's imagination within Eiko's when
Itsuko visualizes her act of murder presented as the second version
of the Hikagejaya incident. In order to evoke the almost deranged
state in which she finds herself now, Yoshida stresses her eyes
reflecting violent flame. Still in her imagination, Itsuko says: "My
dagger pierced his heart. Can you see the blood pouring out of it
like flowing sand? His eyes ceased to blink, and his lips lost their
color. . . . Ōsugi died, and so did my love when I stabbed him. . . ."

The scene of Itsuko's murder is now visually dramatized: we see
Ōsugi staggering, stabbed through the heart. Noe, who shares
Itsuko's imagination, cries: ". . . A gentle dead face. . . . The eyes,
which gazed only at me, cannot see any more. . . . I am going to
follow him in death. . . ."

When we emerge from Itsuko's reverie, we find Ōsugi still alive.
He asks Noe if she is going to follow him even though she knows
that she will be killed. Noe answers that precisely because she
knows that he will be killed, she would like to share his life. Itsuko,
still in her reverie, interrupts and asks Noe what the dead man,

Ōsugi, has said. Noe answers that he has told Itsuko good-bye. Thereupon, we see a close-up of the dagger. We do not know yet why Yoshida has suddenly presented the dagger this way. Only in the light of what happens in the subsequent scene do we realize that the close-up indicates Noe's determination to kill Ōsugi.

The following scene is a woman's argument. Itsuko and Noe each tries to claim the victory in the prolonged battle over Ōsugi. Here, Itsuko's recollection of the second version of the Hikageyaja incident, and the third version of the incident, both in Eiko's imagination, are so closely interacted as to make the dramatic action confusing. Noe cries: "The game is now over. Ōsugi is still alive. When you could not stab him, I knew exactly what I should do. I saw the future at that moment." In spite of Itsuko's protest that Ōsugi is now dead, that she cannot stab a dead person, Noe stabs him in the neck. Blood splashes on to the *tatami* floor suddenly projected on the screen. Ōsugi is now lying on it.

When the scene shifts, to our surprise, Ōsugi is now kneeling. The ensuing conversation among Ōsugi, Noe, and Itsuko resolves the two women's final choices of action in response to the central problem. Here we recognize that Itsuko's motive for free love has not been grounded in idealism but has served as a tool for gratifying her ego.

On the contrary, Noe has recognized that real sexual freedom can be attained only by cutting off her attachment to any particular man. However, when she became involved with Ōsugi, she fell victim to her female instinct. Rationally she admitted the principle of free love but, as her relationship with him grew deeper, she realized that she was competing with two other women for his love. The only way out of her dilemma was to eliminate Ōsugi. She expresses her sense of emotional quandary and resolution this way:

> When you passed through me one day, I was hurt but at the same time I knew what freedom was. I found myself become prisoner of your love. Therefore, this time I had to pass through you trying to be freer.

Ōsugi also expresses Noe's final goal of freedom through her liberation from him, when he says: "Noe, you have won my love in competition with two other women, but at the same time the victory meant becoming my wife. . . . You hated to find yourself in that position."

Our intellectual involvement in the film's action up to this point has been rather intense. However, at the very end of this section

that tension is broken by a touch of a slapstick. Itsuko exclaims that
Ōsugi has died, and appeals to him to say something. Ōsugi opens
his eyes slightly and says: "What do you want a dead person to say?
Call a doctor immediately." This touch of perversity breaks the
spell; and worse, we suspect that Yoshida has engaged us in a mind-
boggling attempt to make sense of three versions of a complex
attempt at homicide—only to deride our efforts.

But we are not given time to recover our poise. The scene shifts
back to the present day. This time we find Eiko and Wada near a
soccer field, discussing the outcome of the Hikagejaya incident. It
is through their conversation that Yoshida tries to offer some clarity
to the homicidal attempt at Hikagejaya and thus to ease our "critical" uneasiness earlier aroused. Wada informs Eiko that Ōsugi was
not stabbed to death in the incident. Faithful to her versions of the
incident, Eiko asks him why Itsuko turned herself into the police
even though she did not kill Ōsugi. Wada attempts to explain
Itsuko's action: Noe committed the imaginary murder of Ōsugi at
Hikagejaya. In order to prevail over Noe in reality and impress
Ōsugi with her love for him, Itsuko claimed herself to be his mur-
deress. Then Wada dismisses Eiko's sustained imaginary acitivity
as meaningless, claiming that the triangular relationship, which
caused Itsuko to turn herself into the police, might not even have
existed. He suddenly runs toward the camera, leaving Eiko alone.

We are again transported into Eiko's imaginary creation of
Ōsugi's and Noe's final death. In this section the past and the
present dynamically intertwine as Eiko puts herself back in the
Taishō period to witness the murder of Ōsugi and Noe. Yoshida
first presents three corpses—Ōsugi's, Noe's, and a boy's.[14] They
are arranged in a circle, heads to the center like petals of a flower.
Against the background of solitary flute music suitable as a kind of
"eulogy," the camera moves away from the corpses. Next, Ōsugi,
Noe, and the boy are standing, and we realize the dynamic nature
of Eiko's imagination, which cannot be rationalized. As Eiko approaches them, they are turned back to corpses, as if to imply that
it is Eiko's difficult task to derive a significant meaning from their
death.

Throughout this scene Yoshida keeps the camera still and drastically limits the characters' physical movement. By so doing, he lets
us feel Eiko's intense concentration upon her imagination, through
which she tires to give some meaning to the massacre. At the end of
this scene, Eiko speaks in a low voice to Noe's corpse: "Noe, do you
know who massacred you? Do you understand?" Then, we recall

the earlier remark made by Ōsugi: "I danced amid the cherry blossoms in early March. . . ." The recollection of this traditional symbol_once more convinces us the dramatic yet fleeting love between Ōsugi and Noe.

All of a sudden, the romantic and elegiac mood changes, and we confront Unema's studio where films are hung like a number of poles to create a very bleak atmosphere. Unema walks across the screen into a pile of rolls of film. The next moment, we see his feet hanging in the air. A shot of the ceiling, from which the rolls of film are hung, conveys a sense of a barren suicide attributable to ennui. When the phrase, "I danced amid the cherry blossoms in early March . . . ," is repeated, we immediately see a striking contrast between the Taishō lovers' dramatic death and Unema's solitary one: a motif that Yoshida has kept exploring thoughout the film. Here again, Yoshida urges a contrast. Ōsugi in his thirties died for his belief; revolution through free love. Unema, a commercial film director also in his thirties, kills himself only to be free from the impoverishment of contemporary love. Ironically, he has to "tie" film around his neck to relieve himself from the burden of living.

In the following scene, the past now encroaches on the present in the contemporary setting as Yoshida presents Wada, Eiko, Ōsugi, Itsuko, and Noe together. Eiko is taking a picture of the Taishō figures. She is using a camera that seems old enough to have been made during the Taishō period. Together with the sound of the shutter, magnesium burns up into a flare. When Eiko says, "Thank you," the camera is static and focuses on the characters who have been lined up for the picture. We recapitulate what has happened to them in the film. After a blackout, we see the dark studio and the entrance on the right side of the screen. Eiko and Wada open the door and go out. The door closes itself. When another blackout is projected, we realize that Eiko and Wada have left the world of imagination and that we have ended our tour of the interacting past and present captured through Eiko's imagination.

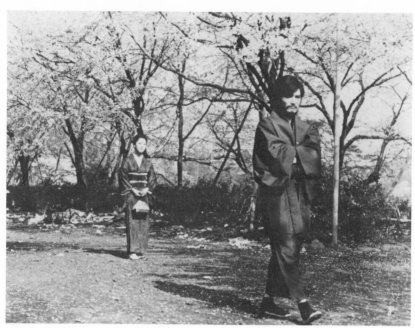

Eros plus Massacre (1969). Ōsugi (Toshiaki Hosokawa) and Noe (Mariko Okada).

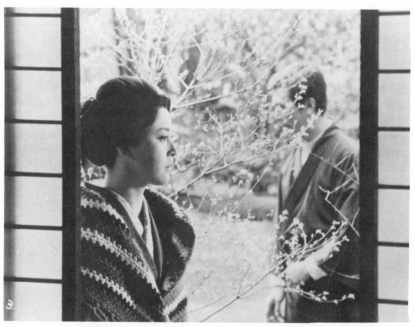

Eros plus Massacre (1969). Noe (Mariko Okada) and her husband (Etsushi Takahashi).

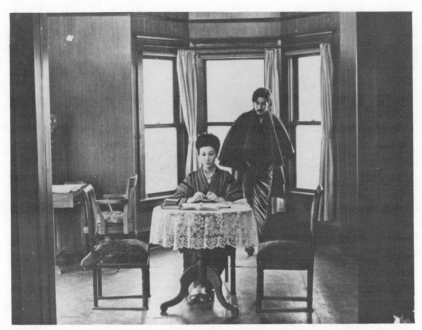

Eros plus Massacre (1969). Ōsugi (Toshiaki Hosokawa) and Itsuko (Yūko Kusunoki).

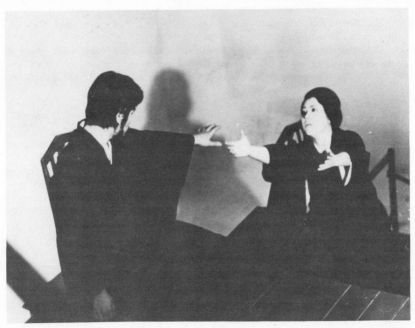

Eros plus Massacre (1969). Ōsugi (Toshiaki Hosokawa) and Noe (Mariko Okada).

NOTES

1. Speaking of the achievement made by Yoshida and Ōshima, representatives of the Japanese *nouvelle vague* movement, Kenji Iwamoto makes the following comment: "Logic and imagination, i.e., conception and the sense of space which bolsters conception—these two elements helped Ōshima and Yoshida to create a conceptual world entirely different from what which the French *Nouvelle Vague* directors formed in their works." See *Nihon Eigashi* [The History of Japanese Cinema] in *Sekai no Eiga Sakka* [Film Directors of the World], (Tokyo: Kinema Jumpo, 1976), 31:220–21.

2. Tadao Satō "*Hakuchi to Ikiru no Sakuhin Kōzō*" [The Structure of *The Idiot* and *Ikiru*,] in *Kurosawa Akira Eiga Taikei* [The Complete Works of Akira Kurosawa] (Tokyo: Kinema Jumpō, 1971), 6:184–85.

3. Quoted by Hiroshi Sekine in "Yoshida Yoshishige no Sekai" [The World of Yoshishige Yoshida], in *Sekai no Eiga Sakka: Shinoda Masahiro: Yoshida Yoshishige* [Film Directors of the World: Masahiro Shinoda: Yoshishige Yoshida] (Tokyo: Kinema Jumpō, 1971), 10:166.

4. When the film was first released in France prior to its release in Japan, it was three and a half hours long. When it was first shown in Japan at the Art Theatre, it was presented in a cut version of two hours and forty-five minutes. The deletion was due to the protest made by Ichiko Kamichika, then a member of the Diet, who was supposed to be the model for Itsuko Masaoka, one of Ōsugi's lovers. As she threatened to sue Yoshida for violation of privacy should the film be released in an unabridged version, Yoshida was forced to cut a number of scenes centered around Itsuko.

5. Tadao Satō, *Nūberu Bāgu Igo: Jiyū o Mezasu Eiga* [After the *Nouvelle Vague*: Films for Freedom] (Tokyo: Chūō Kōron, 1976), p. 146.

6. *Sekai no Eiga Sakka: Shinoda Masahiro: Yoshida Yoshishige* [Film Directors of the World: Masahiro Shinoda: Yoshishige Yoshida], p. 218.

7. Noël Burch, *To the Distant Observer: Form and Meaning in the Japanese Cinema* (Berkeley: University of California Press, 1979), pp. 348–49.

8. The original uncut version shows Unema's lovemaking with Megumi, in which he assumes the father image as well as the child image in order to help her to regress into childhood and also progress into motherhood. Only through her imaginary metamorphosis can she be fulfilled sexually.

9. Ōsugi and Noe were killed by a captain of the military police.

10. Yoshishige Yoshida and Masahiro Yamada, "*Erosu purasu Gyakusatsu*" [Eros plus Massacre], *Āto Shiatā* [Art Theatre] 75:74.

11. Kamichika Ichiko, upon whom Itsuko was modeled, stabbed Ōsugi in the actual Hikagejaya incident, but he was able to save his life.

12. Tadao Satō and Kyōichirō Nanbu, *Nihon Eiga Hyakusen* [One Hundred Selections of Japanese Cinema] (Tokyo: Akita Shoten, 1973), p. 234.

13. Ibid.

14. According to Yoshida, the boy is Sōichi Tachibana, who was killed together with Ōsugi. See "*Erosu purasu Gyakusatsu*" [Eros plus Massacre], p. 80.

PART 6
STORY

10

A Basic Narrative Mode in Yasujirō Ozu's *Tokyo Story*

Simplicity is a word one might use to characterize most of the fifty-four films that Ozu has made since his first film in 1927. Unfortunately, Ozu's simplicity many not be so readily grasped by Western audiences who are unacquainted with Japanese cultural traditions and life-styles. A good example of Japanese simplicity that requires a cultural "footnote" is the famous garden of Ryōanji Temple, which consists of five clusters of rocks arranged in a court-yard or raked sand. This garden offers a classic instance of simplic-ity-as-complexity. The same quality is precisely what makes Ozu "the most Japanese of all directors."[1]

The basis of this simplicity in Ozu's films begins with the simply patterned story that he prefers. It may be useful to approach this important constituent by way of Donald Richie's classification of narrative progression in a film or novel according to three types: anecdote, story, and plot.[2]

The anecdotal narrative, as its name suggests, is the shortest possible account of an event. A number of Godard's films are made up of an accumulation of anecdotes. The story narrative gives events the traditional expansion into a beginning, a middle, and an end. Similarly, the plot narrative arranges events in some order—usually chronological—the difference being one of emphasis; the story emphasizes *what* has happened whereas the plot emphasizes *why* something has happened. An example of this difference can be found in films like Ichikawa's *Conflagration* [Enjō, 1958] and *Odd Obsession* [Kagi, 1959], both of which are heavily plotted. In con-trast, as Donald Richie explains, Ozu's films are storylike:

Just as Ozu's illustrations of his theme are few, so his stories, compared to the majority of those found in full-length films, are slight. A précis of an Ozu film (e.g., daughter lives with father and does not want to marry; she later discovers that his plan to marry again was but a ruse, accomplished for the sake of her future happiness) sounds like too little upon which to base a two-hour film. Any Ozu story, however, is in a way pretext. It is not the story that Ozu wants to show so much as the way his characters react to what happens in the story, and what patterns these relations create. Ozu used progressively simpler stories with each succeeding film, and he rarely availed himself of plot. In the later films the story is little more than anecdote.[3]

What is intriguing about Ozu's films is the way he combines such "simple" thematic and stylistic elements in a story line with such rich effect. Ozu continually returns to a theme that seems peculiarly his: the life of the middle-class Japanese family, and he tells us how the relationships of its members are affected by events in their daily lives. As Donald Richie notes, events in Ozu's films lead typically to the dissolution of the family: "The daughter gets married and leaves the father or the mother alone; the parents go off to live with one of the children; a mother or a father dies. . . ."[4]

Significantly, Ozu stresses the effect of domestic turbulence on individual family members rather than its cause. Incidents of everyday life are used to reveal the nature of various characters gradually, as they act and react.

This emphasis on story rather than plot is easy for Japanese audiences to understand. Ozu's films show everday Japanese life as it is lived. Thus, a viewer in Japan might well say: "I understand that old man's feelings. He is just like me." Another would say: "I feel for the daughter. I was once in the same situation."

Given this strong attachment to familiar scenes and events, Ozu is free to make the most of very simple means. The tempo of his films is leisurely, even slow. His view is quite literally "on the level," the camera typically being fixed at the eye level of a person sitting on a Japanese *tatami* mat. He uses only the three standard shots: long, medium, and close-up. As might be expected, the medium shot is the basic unit of his style and close-ups, even when they are used, are never overly large. There is no waste in the alignment of characters and scenery is presented with an austere formal symmetry and delicate selectiveness that is reminiscent of Japanese brush painting. Sequences tend to open with a rather formal patterning: a cut from an empty exterior to an empty hallway to an empty room that the character enters.[5] Moreover, these formal arragements have much to do with shaping the theme of individual films as the Japanese critic Shinichi Morino points out:

> The coherent form—"an appropriate form of expression which corresponds to the theme of the film"—is not prepared by Ozu; rather, he develops the theme to make it correspond to the symmetry of form. This creative method is a decisive starting point for the appreciation of Ozu's films.[6]

Morino, is referring to the classical dichotomy of form and content. However, in the film as finished product as opposed to product in process, the two are scarcely to be separated; rather, they must be seen as synergistically reinforcing one another to create a harmonious, "artistic" whole.

Tokyo Story [Tokyo Monogatari, 1953], which is often cited as one of Ozu's finest pieces, illuminates the close interaction of these three elements. Despite the simplicity of its story and theme and the economy of its cinematography, the film is complex in ways that Japanese audiences find immediately available, given their intimate knowledge of the cultural milieu which Ozu presents so skillfully. For example, Ozu, the scriptwriter of most of his films, has a masterly way with nuances of meaning and subtle ironies conveyed through the Japanese language itself, and in dialogue. Sometimes a world of meaning is conveyed in little more than a monosyllable spoken by a character. The father in *Tokyo Story* is a famous instance of this "hinting eloquence." Gestures, too, even the most insignificant ones, are apt to portray shades of feeling that cannot be in plain words. The same can be said of "commonplace" views of landscape and characters intercut, charged with philosophical overtones and emotive qualities. One might say that Ozu can and does count on a rich intuitive response from his Japanese audiences. Non-Japanese audiences, who are not steeped in Japanese culture, are apt to miss a myriad of cues, and this discussion of story, theme, and cinematography in *Tokyo Story* is intended to provide some insight into the method of this masterly director.

Tokyo Story was inspired by Leo McCarey's *Make Way for Tomorrow.* The story is a simple three-part tale that focuses on the parents' relationships with their children. The first, and shortest, section of the story, which is set in the little town of Onomichi, shows an old couple (Shūkichi and Tomi) preparing for their trip to Tokyo. The middle section covers their reunion there with their two married children and the widow of their second son. Shūkichi and Tomi experience disillusionment first, with the sort of life that their children have made for themselves in the vast metropolis, and second, with the way their children treat them. The only kindness that they receive comes from their widowed daughter-in-law Noriko. The third section, again set in Onomichi, depicts Tomi's death. The children are called to her deathbed and hurry away after the funeral. Again, it is the daughter-in-law who stays behind to see the old father settled in. Then, she, too must return to Tokyo, leaving him alone with his youngest daughter Kyōko.

As the film's action progresses, the individual characters are more and more illuminated through their reactions to serious and trivial incidents in their daily lives. The cinematic action presented in each section of the story works its way toward the final coda implying the specific world view connected with the traditional Japanese concept of *mujō* (ephemerality of all earthly phenomena).

The central problem that *Tokyo Story* unfolds is "How should one come to terms with the dissolution of a family and, ultimately, with its epitome, death?" Revolving around this central problem are three alternative solutions.

The first, represented by Shūkichi, Tomi, and Noriko, is a calm, resigned acceptance of these human conditions as necessary to our existence. This choice is made by those who possess both compassion and, sensitivity—common emotional traits of Ozu's major characters. Though inwardly affected by separation of the family, they are outwardly calm in the face of inevitable change.

The second alternative, represented by the three older Hirayama children (Kōichi, Shige, and Keizō), is an indifferent, prosaic acceptance of these human conditions. Lacking compassion and sensitivity, they regard the separation of the family as just another inconsequential fact of life.

The youngest child of the Hirayama family, Kyōko, represents the third stance—refusal to accept the dissolution of the family as a manifestation of the irreversible progression of time. Young and inexperienced, Kyōko claims that each family member should attempt to shore up the weakening family solidarity. This last stance, however, is not as distinct an issue as the other two are.

It is not until the middle section of the story that we come to perceive the central problem of the film. *Tokyo Story*, like other Ozu films, does not present a dynamic conflict among these three choices. Rather, we see them co-existing in a complementary way. Although we encounter a mild friction among them toward the end of the middle section and in the final section of the story, these choices are never really seen in opposition to each other, or brought to a resolution.

The first section of the story, the short prelude to the more intense action in the middle, focuses on Shūkichi and Tomi's busy preparation for their trip to Tokyo. Despite its brevity, the scene is rich in significance. The opening shot establishes the geographic location to which the film returns at the end. It is the city of Onomichi, on a morning in early July, as evidenced by the joyous morning markets opened along the street near the ocean. We see a big stone lantern against the background of the ocean. The static ocean and lantern scene quickly cuts back to a motion of a commuter train running through the town. As early as this scene we see a fine example of Ozu's artistry in the equipoise between the static and the mobile. The city spreads from the ocean up the mountainside. We now see the temple, which is later reintroduced as the site of Tomi's funeral. After capturing several schoolchildren walking along a street on the mountainside, the camera moves to the interior of the Hirayamas' house to present the empty hallway and then the couple in their room. This quick transition from exterior to interior to human figures is thematically significant because it reveals the basic philosophical relationship between man and his surroundings that is inherent in Ozu's films. From a basic understanding that man and all the earthly phenomena are mutable, the Japanese develop a keen affinity for their surroundings, of which nature is an integral part.[7] Hence, this rapid sequence already implies man's oneness with his environment as a source of his internal peace, a notion the later cinematic action reinforces. The rest of the beginning section of the story focuses on Shūkichi and Tomi happily engaged in packing their luggage. Their youngest child, Kyōko, a schoolteacher who still lives with them, comes out from the kitchen.

KYOKO: Here is your lunch. I'm leaving now.
(She puts her own lunch box in her bag.)
TOMI: If you're busy at school you don't need to come see us off, you know.
KYOKO: I think I'll have time. It's the physical-education period.
SHUKICHI: We'll see you later at the station then.
KYOKO: I've put the tea in the thermos, Mother.
TOMI: All right.
KYOKO: I'll be going then.[8]

From what little Ozu has presented of their conversation, we

already sense a congenial harmony between the youngest daughter
and her parents and their mutual caring for each other. After
Kyōko is gone, Shūkichi and Tomi start looking for an air pillow,
which the husband claims his wife put away in her luggage. The
wife starts looking into her things. A next-door neighbor passes by
the window of their room. The neighbor's appearance is an indispensable part of Ozu's formalism: repetition or parallelism. The
neighbor appears at the same site in the last sequence of the film.
The neighbor says that both Shūkichi and Tomi must be really
contented to have such a fine son and daughter living in Tokyo.
Shūkichi replies complacently yet modestly (in a traditional Japanese manner): "Well, they are just ordinary children. . . ." His
remark is meant to be double irony in light of subsequent developments: what Shūkichi really means is that he believes that
their grown-up children are wonderful people. They really are,
contrary to their parents' expectation; they turn out indeed to be
"just ordinary children," to their parents' disappointment. After
the neighbor refers to the fine weather, a most ordinary topic of
conversation and therefore another "everyday cue" typical of Ozu,
she wishes the couple bon voyage and leaves them. The camera
focuses again on the couple, who are still looking for the air pillow.
Shūkichi finally says: "I've found it." Tomi responds: "You have
found it, haven't you?" Their action and dialogue, tinged with a
Hiroshima dialect, illuminate their characters: We sense a conjugal
happiness that has lasted into old age; an affection for their children; and a harmony within themselves and with the external
world.

The middle section of the story takes us to Tokyo where we see
how the old couple's initial expectations of their own children are
betrayed and how they cope with the dissolution of their family. At
the same time we also see how Kōichi and Shige unintentionally
work against family unity and how Noriko affirms the traditional
parents–daughter-in-law relationship. In this section, too, we
gradually perceive the individual characters' natures and personalities through trivial incidents in their lives and little remarks
they make.

As in the first section of the story, this middle section often
presents Ozu's formalistic use of transitions from place to place. He
cuts from the exterior to the empty interior of the house and then to
human figures inside. For example, in strong contrast to the peaceful scenic landscape of Onomichi in the first section, this section
opens with chimneys sticking out against a gray sky, revealing the

ugly aspects of industrial Tokyo and foreshadowing the old couple's disillusionment with the metropolis. Gradually the scene narrows. We see the station located in the vicinity of Kōichi's house and an empty lot at a street corner where a sign reads: "Hirayama Clinic—General Practitioner and Pediatrician." A shot of the doctor's office inside Kōichi's house, in turn, is succeeded by an empty corridor leading to the second floor. After a symmetrical presentation of empty exterior and interior—a typical Ozu procedure—we see for the first time Kōichi's wife, Fumiko, in a room on the second floor. She is busily cleaning what appears to be her children's room. The study desk has been moved into a corner of the corridor so that the room will serve as a guestroom during the old couple's visit. When Fumiko's elder son, Minoru, comes home, he complains about this arrangement. In this short scene, Ozu reveals something essential about Fumiko's basic nature: her insensitivity to others. When Minoru asks where he can study, Fumiko nonchalantly tells him that he can study anywhere. When he follows her around, asking her again where he can study, she tells him crossly not to pester her since he does not study very much anyway and has no reason to fuss.

The following scene brings the old couple, their two children (Kōichi and Shige), and the widow Noriko together. Here too Ozu shows us much in little. First, we see Kōichi and Fumiko greeting Shūkichi and Tomi in their living room. After a succession of events outside the room, Ozu cuts to the living room to show us Shige, the couple's elder daughter joining the party. Again, a succession of events outside the room follows and Ozu cuts back into the room to present Noriko joining the party. This formalism makes us feel a kind of tension in the formality between the couple and children. However, when Ozu moves in with a series of medium shots to show us Shūkichi, Tomi, and Noriko greeting one another, we sense the warm relationship between parents and daughter-in-law, despite the formality of their behavior. That warmth is reinforced by the repetitive use of point-of-view and reverse-angle shots. Shūkichi and Tomi are aligned together, sitting opposite Noriko. First a frontal medium shot of Shūkichi is presented, then quickly taken over by a frontal medium shot of the smiling Noriko, which, in turn, yields to a frontal medium shot of the smiling Tomi. After two more medium shots of Shūkichi and Noriko, respectively Ozu presents a medium shot of the three together. Finally, there follows a crosscutting between Noriko and Shūkichi. By careful employment of these frontal medium shots from the eye level of a person sitting on the *tatami* mat, Ozu invites us to empathize with them. For example, when he presents Shūkichi greeting Noriko, we share Noriko's viewpoint. When Noriko speaks to her father-in-law, we assume his perspective and watch her, and so forth. This movement back and forth between parents and daughter-in-law builds our appreciation of the congenial relationship between them.

In discussing Ozu's systemic in *That Night's Wife*, Noël Burch makes an interesting comment on the director's reverse-field setup:

> . . . by undermining the verisimilitude of face-to-face reverse-field situations, Ozu challenged the *principle of the inclusion of the viewer in the diegesis* as invisible, transparent relay in the communion of two characters. Once the spectator is unconsciously obliged to rectify with each new shot-change his mental position with respect to the players, the trap of participation no longer functions in quite the same way.[9]

Burch goes on to refer to the comment made by Satō that "Ozu's characters speak to themselves rather than to their partners."[10]

However, Ozu's films do urge us to distinguish between aesthetic and emotional distances. In this sequence of *Tokyo Story*, for example, the fixed position of the camera and the symmetrical alignment of the three characters create a kind of aesthetic distance: we are given the impression that we are watching their action as invited guests sitting in their drawing room or attending the tea ceremony. Furthermore, the fact that none of the three, taken in medium shot, is looking straight into the camera's eyes, and hence, into our eyes, while they are smiling, also augments a sense of ceremonial remoteness. This sense is similar to what we feel, looking at a smiling mask. However, this aesthetic (formal) distance is heavily offset by our emotional involvement with the three characters. The kind of world that they offer us is an extension of our daily lives, and because of this affinity, we are drawn into the characters' minds. We also come to consider their gesture in averting the camera's eyes as a manifestation of a typical Japanese character trait—shyness—and we feel that they are just like us. Thus, our emotional involvement is the basic rhetorical stance that is sustained throughout the film.

In this sequence, we gain insight into the personality of the old couple's married children, not from the scenes where they are with their parents but from those in which the parents are absent. When, in the kitchen, Shige and Kōichi make a casual remark that sukiyaki is good enough for their parents and that they should not go out of their way to serve something additional like *sashimi*, we learn something important about their attitude. They have not seen Shūkichi and Tomi for a long time, yet they are too economy-minded to entertain them with a feast. Furthermore, by contrasting two images that might easily escape our attention—the cheap pickled seaweeds and cookies, which Shige bought for the entire party at a nearby shop, and the box of very nice cookies Noriko bought in spite of her tight budget—Ozu shows us a clear distinction between Shige's and Noriko's attitudes toward Shūkichi and Tomi.

As early as the beginning of this middle section of the story, Ozu has already verbally presented the old couple's disillusionment with both the city of Tokyo and Kōichi's success as a medical doctor. After introducing the empty guestroom with Minoru's desk still outside, Ozu shows Shūkichi and Tomi entering it to sit on the *futon* (sleeping mattress). They talk. Tomi says that she expected Kōichi's office to be in a more agreeable area than this dingy neighborhood. Shūkichi responds that though his son wanted to open his clinic in a better place, he just has to be satisfied with the office he has now. They become pensive. The frontal medium shots hitherto employed suddenly change into profiles. Though they do not speak now, their profiles speak for them, expressing their resigned acceptance of the way things are in spite of their disillusionment.

With the chimneys reintroduced as a pivotal point, the scene cuts to Shige's beauty shop. Through a brief banal conversation between Shige and her husband, we are again exposed to her attitude toward her parents. When her husband suggests that he take them to a restaurant upon their arrival, Shige tells him not to bother. From this point on, the film intensifies its portrayal of the theme of filial ingratitude.

At both Kōichi's and Shige's homes, Shūkichi and Tomi do not receive the kind of welcome they expected. Kōichi, who was supposed to take his parents out sightseeing, cannot do so as he is called out for an emergency. Next, at Shige's place, we see both Shige and her husband too busy to take a little time out for sightseeing with the old couple. Both Tomi and Shūkichi are left alone in the beauty shop. The only place to go is the public bathhouse where Shige's husband takes the couple. The inconsiderate daughter even gives her mother some mending to do.

Without fuss or complaint about their children's pursuit of their busy lives, Shūkichi and Tomi face a failure of family structure. They sadly resign themselves to the fact that each child has his own family and goal to pursue and that they cannot recapture the moment of keen parent-child kinship which they knew in the past. In a very subtle way Ozu captures the solitude and loneliness experienced by the old couple. For example, after presenting Tomi and her grandchild playing in an empty lot, he cuts back to the interior of Kōichi's house where Shūkichi sits alone, moving a fan slowly— a gesture typical of so many Ozu characters. This is a sudden moment of illumination to us, as a sense of quiescent, sad resignation is transmitted to us as strongly as the immediacy of our experience. Significantly, Ozu closes this shot with a fade—a technique that is very rarely used in his films—in order to add a elegiac texture to the old man's plight.

In contrast, both Shige and Kōichi view the dissolution of the family with notable calm. They take for granted a rift that, however self-consciously "modern," is still very troubling to Japanese audiences. Shige and Kōichi reason drily that they have their own lives to lead—and so do their parents. Their insensitivity is quickly apparent, and important as a breach and barrier between them and their parents. Shūkichi and Tomi cannot communicate their feelings about this tragic rift; and in any case, their children would be too unsympathetic to listen. For example, when Shige sees Tomi ready to go to the public bathhouse, she, still busily occupied with her customer, yells at Tomi to wear a dirty pair of her own *geta* (clogs) to the place. The mother takes her daughter's thoughtless slight in stride. However, we, the audience, take it very much to heart. Ozu manages through this trivial incident to give us a "direct" sense of Shige's ignorant want of tenderness toward the aged in general.

One of the major events in this section of the story is the old couple's trip to Atami, a hot spring resort. Too busy to take care of their parents, Shige and Kōichi decide to send them to a cheap Japanese inn at Atami for a few days of recreation. This is their expedient means for releasing themselves from the burden of personally entertaining their parents. The hot spring scene bears thematic significance because it not only exposes the nature of the children's attitudes toward their parents but also reveals the way the aged couple face their own lives, in which changes are inevitable. Unaware of their children's real intention, Shūkichi and Tomi, dressed in the summer kimonos *(yukata)* furnished by the inn, enjoy a moment of relaxation. At the same time they feel somewhat guilty about the unnecessary expense that Kōichi and Shige have been put to. Shūkichi, looking at the sea that stretches beneath the

window of their room, says in a monotonous voice: "The quiet sea
. . ." Tomi responds: "Yes. . . ."

Through the banal experience of the old couple, we have already
become aware that Shūkichi and Tomi try to face the progression
of time and its concomitant changes in life, in accord with the
traditional view of life, its cyclic pattern, according to which man is
born and dies. Thus, when Ozu cuts to the exterior of the inn and
presents a single shot of the ocean and the island, this single shot
again marks for us the illuminating moment of the couple's internal
peace: the calm serene sea, the epitome of Mother Nature, and an
index of the fertile life force envelops the island and externalizes
their harmony with Nature.

The following scene shows the commercialization, which has
vulgarized this resort town, and which in this film is portrayed as a
threat to the traditional values of close family life. The serenity of
the inn where the couple are staying vanishes with the arrival of a
horde of fun-seeking office workers. They stay up all night, playing
Mah-jongg, while street singers noisily sing popular songs outside.
Later we learn from two maids' casual conversation just what kinds
of guests the inn has been receiving lately. A newlywed couple who
stayed in the inn were not respectable; while the husband was
already up, the bride stayed in bed, puffing a cigarette. Amid the
noise assaulting their room, Shūkichi and Tomi cannot sleep, even
though they have been in bed for some time. They do not rage
against the noise, nor do they verbally complain. All they do is
sigh, with their emotions well under control. Watching the couple,
we are not uneasy at their feelings but almost smile at their somewhat naive calm—an attitude derived from the aged wisdom that is
very common among the traditional Japanese.

Noriko, whose husband has been dead for eight years, also represents the choice of resigned acceptance of the dissolution of the
family clearly manifested by her husband's death. However, it is
her unconscious exercise of gratitude, reverence, and compassion
for her aged parents-in-law that mitigates their otherwise too stark
awareness of the dissolution of the bond between them and their
three children (Keizō, Kōichi, and Shige). Unlike Shige and, to a
certain extent, Kōichi's wife, Noriko still retains traits of a traditional Japanese woman—respect for the aged, sensitivity to the
feelings of others, and acceptance of her own suffering—which
Ozu's films depict as being gradually threatened by the modernization of Japan.

The middle of the story presents three important scenes which

reveal the solidarity between Noriko and the old couple. The first
takes place in the early part of the middle section. Noriko is asked
by the demanding Shige to take a day off from her work to take
Shūkichi and Tomi on a sightseeing tour of Tokyo. Noriko does so
willingly. After presenting the curious couple and Noriko on the
sightseeing tour, Ozu takes us to the interior of Noriko's shabby
apartment. Shūkichi and Tomi gaze at the picture of Noriko's deceased husband, Shōji, placed on the shelf. Meanwhile, Noriko
serves Shūkichi sake, his favorite drink. There is repeated cutting
among the faces of Noriko and the elderly couple, all taken in a
close-up, while their conversation goes on. These close-ups (never
large ones) articulate Shūkichi's almost childlike delight at the treat
of the sake, Tomi's relaxation, which is impossible at her own two
children's homes, and Noriko's satisfaction.

The second scene involves Tomi's overnight stay at Noriko's
place, which affirms the mother–daughter-in-law bond as their last
union before Tomi's death. Prior to introducing this scene, Ozu
presents the old couple's unexpected return from Atami caused by
their discomfort with the atmosphere of the resort. The transition
from Atami to Tokyo is again presented by three shots of empty
landscapes, a typical Ozu style: a long shot of the island on the
ocean, which the couple earlier watched while sipping tea at their
Japanese inn, then a medium shot of the island, and finally a long
shot of the chimneys, a recurrent image, which earlier also served
as a pivotal point for a shift in location. These three shots resolve in
a shot of Shige's beauty shop where she is busily setting a customer's hair. Shige is surprised to find that her parents have returned
from their trip so soon. Again we are exposed to her lack of consideration. When the customer asks her who the old couple are, she
is too embarrassed to acknowledge them. She says that they are
acquaintances, just in from the country. Ozu concludes this incident with subtle irony. First, her parents do not hear Shige's remark, and this spares them from being hurt by her insensitivity.
Second, Shūkichi and Tomi assume that they will be able to relax
more at her place than at the inn. But their expectation is betrayed.
Shige tells them that she did not want them to return so early, as
she was planning to run a workshop at her place in the evening.
Shige's lack of empathy saves her from feeling guilty.

Ozu then cuts from Shige's house to a corner of Ueno Park.
Here, the couple decide that since Noriko's place is too small to
accommodate both of them, Tomi will stay with Noriko and
Shūkichi will visit an old acquaintance from Onomichi. It is time

for them to leave. Ozu then presents a long shot of the couple walking together to the town. They do not say anything, but this single shot speaks for them. It reaffirms the conjugal solidarity, which we have encountered in their earlier conservation: "Tokyo is such a big place. . . ." "Yes, if you get lost here, I would have to spend the rest of my life looking for you."

Soft violin music on the sound track helps this reaffirmation. This long shot does not evoke a sense of the old couple's harmony with their surroundings; rather, it emphasizes their isolation in the unfamiliar town, especially now that we know that the simple old couple, who have never been separated in their late years, must sleep apart from each other in the huge metropolis.

Next, we enter Noriko's apartment for the second important scene of mutual compassion. Again the scene opens in a typical Ozu manner with a cut from the empty corridor to the inside of the apartment. The shot of the corridor is accompanied by the bong of a clock somewhere, Ozu's favorite metaphor, which establishes the temporal setting for the dramatic action that is to follow. It is midnight. Two quilt beds have already been made, and Noriko is rubbing Tomi's shoulder. To Japanese audiences this familiar scene is the very index of domestic harmony articulating the young's caring for the aged. After Noriko puts the quilt over her, Tomi hesitantly says that, as her mother-in-law, she feels badly that Noriko remains unmarried now that eight years have passed since her husband's death. Noriko smilingly responds that she does not want to remarry, not because she is loyal to her late husband, but because she is more comfortable living alone. Again, we must read between the lines of this conversation. We find in it a genuine mutual compassion as these two women articulate a king of resignation in face of the merciless progression of time.

To conclude this domestic scene, Ozu suddenly introduces a rare moment of emotional outburst in these two women. Tomi, touched by Noriko's deep bond to her parents-in-law, says: "You're such a good person. . . ." Thereupon, Noriko plainly says, "Good night," switches off the light, and creeps into her bed. Tomi is asleep next to her as Ozu cuts to Noriko to present a close-up of her profile. Again, Ozu limits his use of the close-up mostly to the climatic moment of emotion. Our natural response is to feel for Noriko. Her face almost in tears shows not only sympathy for her parents-in-law, who have been ill treated by their married children, but also pity for herself, embittered by her husband's death. Furthermore, this close-up is a prime example of the revelation of the basic nature of Ozu characters, who accept things with sad resignation. Noriko has kept her inner harmony, courageously attempting to overcome a sense of anomie caused by Shōji's death. Ironically, it is Tomi's visit that threatens her inner peace, like a stone disturbing the calm surface of the water. A sense of isolation from her environment and uncertainty about her future is also momentarily crystallized in Noriko's tearful eyes.

The scene the following morning shifts, in a typical Ozu manner, from the deserted street to the empty corridor of Noriko's apartment. Noriko enters the corridor with the dishes she has just washed in the communal kitchen. In this way, we are introduced to the final important scene of solidarity between the mother and daughter-in-law. When Ozu cuts to the inside, Noriko smilingly gives Tomi a small envelope containing money, apologizing for the small amount. Tomi first declines, but finally gives in. This kind little gesture, of which her own daughter, Shige, is incapable, touches Tomi so that her eyes fill with tears. Secretly wiping her tears, Tomi hears Noriko say: "Please come back here again. . . ." Their conversation strikes us as trivial and perfunctory, but it says enough: it emphasizes their deep mutual caring, a rare asset amid encroaching modernization; rare even in the context of traditional society where mother–daughter-in-law friction is a common phenomenon. Furthermore, their conversation foreshadows Tomi's death.

Death plays an important part in uniting the family members. Just as the memories of the late Shōji brings Noriko, Tomi, and Shūkichi together, Tomi's death paves the way for the climactic bonding of father-in-law and daughter-in-law.

In the meantime, we also witness Shūkichi's actions after leaving Tomi. In his recent book, *Transcendental Style in Film: Ozu, Bresson, Dreyer*, Paul Schrader points out the nagging sense of disparity that Ozu's characters experience in their everyday lives. Schrader terms this disparity "an actual or potential disunity between man and his environment which culminates in a decisive action,"[11] which, he thinks, offers a valuable approach to Ozu's major characters. In this film, as well, a sense of disparity exists in Noriko and Shūkichi, not as a discordant element in their consciousness but as subconscious feelings existing alongside resignation in a complementary way. One decisive action, which brings this discordant element out into view, is Noriko's weeping.

Another way in which Ozu's characters cope with this disparity

is through a sudden emotional outburst over sake. A number of
Ozu's films include restaurant or tavern scenes, in which his
characters, getting drunk or quietly sipping sake, reveal their sense
of disunity or anxiety. These scenes are rare moments of character
revelation; we witness a momentary surge of true feelings in characters who, in their daily lives, silently endure a sense of disparity
with calm detachment or with a display of a good sense of humor.

Ever since their arrival in Tokyo, Shūkichi and Tomi confronted
an unfamiliar environment. This is illustrated by the recurrent
image of the ugly industrial chimneys and their grown-up children's attitudes toward them. Capable of sustaining an inner equilibrium, the couple have accepted desertion and discord quietly.

Their state of mind can be most clearly described in the famous
image of the water basin that Junichirō Tanizaki employs in *Some
Prefer Nettles* [*Tade Kū Mushi*]: the static basin filled with the water,
whose surface is calm, but whose balance may tilt at any time.
Somewhere in Shūkichi's mind, a sense of emotional dissatisfaction
is subconciously present, though well under control. However,
there are certain times when his inner peace is threatened. Thus,
when Ozu cuts to a tavern from Noriko's apartment to present
Shūkichi's evening after leaving Tomi, Shūkichi's latent discontent
emerges. Here, we see Shūkichi, Hattori, and Numata, an acquaintance of Shūkichi's. Hattori, having had one drink too many,
is ready to fall asleep.

The ensuing conversation about their sons between Shūkichi and
Numata articulates a sense of disunity that they sometimes find
difficult to accept with resignation, though they try. It also reveals
Shūkichi's "loquacity," in contrast to his earlier almost monosyl-
labic talk:

NUMATA: No, he's a failure. My only son. And I wasn't strong
          enough. I spoiled him. Now you. Your brought up your
          son proper. He has a degree.
SHUKICHI: Nowadays all doctors have to have degrees.
NUMATA: Maybe we expect too much of our children. But they lack
          ambition, they lack real spirit. That is just what I told my
          son. And then he said to me that there are too many people
          in Tokyo and so it's hard to get ahead. What do you think of
          that? Young people today just have no backbone. Where is
          their spirit? (SHUKICHI tries to protest.) Well, I'm a disap-
          pointed man. But you—you couldn't feel that way. You
          must be very satisfied.

SHUKICHI: Of course, I'm not, but—

NUMATA: You see? It's gotten so bad that even you can't be satisfied. Oh, I feel so sad. (Rubs his eyes).

HATTORI: Oh, I just can't drink any more. (Sinks back and closes his eyes again.)

SHUKICHI: Well, when I came up to Tokyo, I was under the impression that my son was doing better than he is. Then I found he's only this little neighborhood doctor . . . so, I know how you feel. I'm just as dissatisfied as you are. But we can't expect too much from our children. Times have changed and we have to face it. That's what I think.

NUMATA: You do?

SHUKICHI: Yes.

NUMATA: There, you see? You too.

SHUKICHI: My son has really changed. But I can't help it. There really are too many people in Tokyo.

NUMATA: I wonder.

SHUKICHI: Well, maybe it's a good thing.

NUMATA: I suppose I should be happy. Nowadays some young men would kill their parents without a thought. Mine at least wouldn't do that. (Laughs.)[12]

A momentary outburst, fueled by their latent dissatisfaction, recedes with their defense of their children. They are capable of looking at their own situations with a sense of humor, and at the same time they can protect their own children with compassion, attributing the effacement of filial loyalty to external forces at work in the city. As in his many other films, Ozu then shows his characters drinking; both Shūkichi and Numata, completely drunk forget about their petty everyday troubles, which weigh them down, and arrive at Shige's house to fall dead asleep on chairs in her beauty shop. Perhaps, here Ozu intends an irony that disappointed parents, like disappointing children, fall short of the best behavior.

The final part of the story, the climax of the film, shifts back to Onomichi. It is in this last section of the story that the widely separated Hirayama family members—Shūkichi and Kyōko in Onomichi, Keizō in Osaka, and Kōichi, Shige, and Noriko in Tokyo—are brought together. This part also opens with Ozu's cinematic norm—two shots of empty settings; one the alley in front of the Hirayamas' house, the other the open corridor inside their house. The camera moves into a room where Tomi is confined to bed, watched by Shūkichi and Kyōko.

After Kyōko leaves the room, we see Shūkichi all alone, sighing, watching Tomi asleep in bed. As if he were talking to himself, he keeps talking to his sleeping wife. Noticing her slight movement, Shūkichi says: "What's the matter? . . . Um. . . . Do you feel warm?" Tomi does not respond, and Shūkichi says that soon all the children will come to her, repeatedly adding: "Surely, you'll recover." This repeated phrase is Shūkichi's own expression of self-assurance. His almost monotonous speech and almost gestureless pose reveal his deep sorrow, which we unhesitantly share, over his wife's approaching death. At the same time we sense the presence of the subtle, unbreakable conjugal bond, which has permeated their lives. Regardless of the dissolution of the family, which they have encountered since their children's marriages, they have nonetheless felt lucky. Witnessing this scene, we remember the conversation they had at Keizō's boardinghouse in Ōsaka, their last stop on their way back to Onomichi:

SHUKICHI: But I'm surprised at how children change. Shige, now—she used to be much nicer before. A married daughter is like a stranger.
TOMI: Koichi's changed too. He used to be such a nice boy.
SHUKICHI: No, children don't live up to their parents' expectations. (They both laugh.) But, if you are greedy then there is no end to it. Let's think that they are better than most.
TOMI: They are certainly better than average. We are fortunate.
SHUKICHI: Yes, fortunate. We should consider ourselves lucky.[13]

We also vividly recall the resigned smile with which Tomi and Shūkichi reassured each other of their good fortune. By now we have been fully convinced that it is their internal serenity and aged wisdom that have led them to accept the breakdown of their family with compassion and resignation. Now, seing Shūkichi talking to Tomi (and to himself), we become aware that he will face his wife's inevitable death with equal resignation, accepting his inability to fight against the flux of time. The camera cuts to the yard to present the flowers swaying in the July breeze from Shūkichi's perspective. The flowers, symbolic of nature's exuberant life force, suggest Shūkichi's wish nonetheless for Tomi's recovery, rather than reinforcing Shūkichi's acceptance of *mujō*.

After Tomi's death, Ozu again cuts to the exterior of the house to show the empty landscape, now charged with meaning. It is dawn. A close-up of the big lantern earlier presented against the ocean is superseded by a long shot of a ship gliding into the harbor. These

two shots are a prime example of Ozu's magnificent juxtaposition of
the static and the mobile, indicating complete harmony between
manmade objects and surrounding nature. Time passes; seasons
change; there is a world of natural events indifferent to human
affairs. Both human affairs and Nature are but insignificant components of the large span of time. This universal law expressed by
these shots of the empty exterior is what Shūkichi, in the face of his
beloved wife's death, must come to accept, and so he does.

Now the camera cuts to the interior of the Hirayama house
where the survivors—Shige, Kōichi, Noriko and Kyōko—are in
mourning, surrounding Tomi, whose face is covered with a white
cloth according to the Japanese custom. As previously stated, death
momentarily unites the family in sorrow. Kyōko keeps wiping her
tears. Shige says: "Human beings are so evanescent. . . ." Nobody
responds, and Shige, wiping her tears, once more says: "She was so
healthy. . . ." Noriko quietly wipes her tears. This momentarily
restored family unity, however, soon dissolves in discord when
Shige's verbosity becomes unbearable to both Noriko's and
Kyōko's sensitivities. Shige claims that Tomi suspected she would
soon die and that that explained the trip to Tokyo. Kōichi monosyl-
labically agrees with her. Shige then impolitely asks Noriko
whether she has brought her funeral dress with her. Hearing
Noriko's negative reply, Shige suggests that both Noriko and
Kyōko must borrow mourning dresses somewhere. Ozu lets her
words reveal Shige's character—ignorance of the dictum that Silence is golden on occasions like this. Furthermore, Ozu treats
Shige ironically in order to emphasize her lack of sensitivity. Shige
says complacently: "Mother died a peaceful death. She died without suffering. . . ." She is completely unaware that her own inconsiderate behavior caused her mother such discomfort when they
were last together.

After the arrival of Keizō, who did not come in time for Tomi's
death, Noriko goes outside to look for Shūkichi, who has been
absent from home for some time. Ozu cuts to Shūkichi standing in
an empty lot on top of a cliff. Noriko approaches him. The following scene, reuniting Noriko and her father-in-law in mutual empathy, anticipates the final dramatization of deep human
compassion that will take place later. When Noriko tells him that
Keizō has arrived, Shūkichi, in turn, tells her that he has seen a
magnificent dawn. Noriko cannot utter a word, her sensitivity
deeply touched by his solitude. He continues: "It will be a hot
today," an expression very common among Ozu's characters.

Shūkichi's frequent reference to nature expresses man's affinity with it, and therefore with man's acceptance of the universal law governing his world: the inevitable progression of time. Shūkichi quietly starts walking home, followed by Noriko. A long shot of the two in perfect concordance with the surrounding scenery subtly externalizes their almost stoic resignation, which makes their serene acceptance of Tomi's death possible.

Now we are initiated into the most dramatic scene of the film, Tomi's funeral. To guide us to the interior of the temple, the site of the funeral, Ozu again uses two shots of empty scenes: first, a close-up of the temple wall; and then a long shot of the entire building. These two shots are accompanied by the sounds of the priests' prayer and the wooden prayer drum coming from inside the main hall. We see Shūkichi and his children sitting in a row in mourning. The filmic composition of this take is an impressive combination of Ozu's aesthetic and thematic concerns; it reveals his formal perfection and at the same time it serves as an adept medium for reinforcing the concept of *mujō* (the mutability of all earthly phenomena) sustained throughout the film. Tomi's survivors, Shūkichi, Kōichi, Shige, Keizō, Noriko, and Kyōko sit diagonally across the screen; each slightly bowing his or her head expressing sorrow. Two pillars inside the main hall—one beside Shūkichi, farthest away, and the other between Noriko and Kyōko sitting closest to the camera—enhance the symmetrical harmony of composition here. This rigid alignment of figures expresses, more effectively than any verbal expression, the constant flow of time, which these survivors solemnly experience at this moment.

In the earlier scenes of the third part of the story, Ozu employed a series of similar compositions to demonstrate the calm with which the survivors watched Tomi confined to bed. As Tadao Satō points out, Tomi's bed is arranged at the lower right of the screen, and her family members, who watch her, sit closer to the left side of the screen, either facing the camera or perpendicular to it. When each person leaves the room and returns, he or she resumes the same sitting position.[14] These shots anticipate, and prepare us for, the final harmonious composition of the funeral take. Concerning Ozu's compositional frame for the funeral scene, Satō says:

> There are many places in this film where the compositional frame shows everyone sitting in the same position facing the same way, and one of the best examples of this is the funeral scene in the main hall of the temple following the mother's death. All of the participants are

sitting in a row, attired in mourning dress, with each one, male and female, young and old, facing the same direction and holding their head at the same angle. And yet one does not get the impression of a military formation with people forced to assume a fixed posture along a straight line. At first glance, it looks completely natural and unposed, but in fact it is a scene in which all the asymmetry and disharmony which inevitably exist in a real situation have been carefully eliminated. It is not a composition of forced totalitarian uniformity, but one of meditation which concentrates people's attention on a single point. Or, better, it is one which makes us imagine that the characters in the story, by concentrating on one thing, have fallen into a state of mind similar to meditation. Then, as to what appears to one in this contemplative state, it is life—endlessly changing and renewing, and the preciousness of time.[15]

In the middle of the ceremony, Keizō suddenly leaves the main hall. The camera cuts to a corner where he sits sadly, staring outside. Next follows a point-of-view shot of the cemetery against the sea in the distance. In its fusion of life and death, this single shot effectively reasserts the cyclic pattern, which man lives unconsciously in his daily life but which he suddenly experiences as a revelation at such a crucial moment as the death of someone in his family. Man's inability to reverse time is clearly manifested in Keizō's remark to Noriko, who comes to inform him that it will soon be his turn to burn incense for his mother. Keizō says that the sounds of the wooden drum give him the impression of his mother's gradually diminishing, and that he is sorry for not having been kind to her while she was alive. After Keizō and Noriko leave the corner, Ozu's camera again captures the cemetery against the distant ocean, this time with an accompaniment of a sutra being chanted. When Ozu's subsequent shot shows the beach swept by the tide, the sense of the human world governed by the cosmic law of mutability becomes consummate in the blending of the fertile and the decayed.

Tomi's death and funeral restore family unity for a short time. However, after the funeral this moment of equilibrium dissolves quite naturally and rapidly. On the second floor of an old restaurant near the ocean, Shūkichi, Kōichi, Shige, Noriko, Keizō and Kyōko are seated at the table sharing their memories of Tomi: the firecrackers which Keizō saw from this very room when he was a child; the spring trips they took with their parents in childhood; and so on. However, as soon as Shūkichi excuses himself for a moment, Shige, Keizō, and Kōichi begin to show, in their own ways, their insensitivity and selfishness. They want to leave as soon as possible; only Noriko agrees to stay behind.

In this last part of the film Ozu continually returns to the ocean image. Sometimes it is obliquely present, as in the restaurant scene, where the water is reflected in a glitter on the ceiling and the room partition (*fusuma*), as if to assert the quiet presence of a vast, transcendent, peaceful force at work in a world stirred, here, by the squalid petty discord of these three children.

Up to this point, Ozu has been careful to confine his comment on the breakup of the Hirayama family to subtle verbal ironies. For example, in the funeral scene Keizō has told Noriko that the wooden drum beating for the service reminds him of his dead mother's gradually shrinking. By and large, Ozu has used these verbal ironies adeptly to incite our wry smile at the three Hirayama children's breach of filial piety and thus to keep us from accepting their attitudes as an extention of ours.

It is during Kyōko's confrontation with Noriko that Ozu brings the three hitherto sustained ways of acceptance to an open yet mild friction for the first time. Kyōko blames Shige, Keizō, and Kōichi for having been so selfish and insensitive to their father. Her anger is directed at Shige especially, since it was she who had the audacity to ask for a memento immediately after Tomi's funeral. At the same time Kyōko declares that she refuses to accept the changes in the Hirayama family, saying that the close parent-child relationship she experienced in her childhood should be maintained even now. She adds, however, that even among mere acquaintances she finds much warmer relationships than she has with her siblings.

Noriko says:

> But, look, Kyōko. At your age I thought as you do. But children do drift away from their parents. A woman has her own life, apart from her parents, when she is Shige's age. She meant no harm, I'm sure. It's only that everyone has to look after himself.[16]

Through Noriko's mouth Ozu seems to defend the attitudes of the accused, and thus to emphasize the relativity of each party's acceptance of the crude reality of the progression of time. During Noriko's talk to Kyōko, we are reminded that Shūkichi, Tomi, and Noriko have faced the dissolution of the Hirayama family with reticent resignation and that compassion can be a source of internal peace, just as sensitivity can result in the occasional emotional outburst. We are also reminded that because of their very lack of those human traits, Kōichi, Shige, and Keizō are not capable of the deeper level of spiritual satisfaction and consequently they are spared internal suffering, too.

In the earlier scenes of Shūkichi and Tomi's visit to Noriko's place and Tomi's overnight stay with her, we have twice witnessed the warm relationship between parents and daughter-in-law. Now we realize that those scenes anticipate a final affirmation of deep-rooted sympathy between father and daughter-in-law. Again, two long shots of empty settings prepare us for this moment of special climatic affinity: the first shows us the room where Kyōko and Noriko have been talking; the second shifts to a hallway. Noriko enters and starts tidying the room. Shūkichi joins her, drying his hands with a towel. Their ensuing conversation becomes more substantial than their previous ones. Beneath its formality and rather dispassionate nature, we detect a deep undercurrent of mutual respect and caring. Noriko tells Shūkichi that she is leaving for Tokyo soon. Shūkichi expresses his gratitude to her for staying with them so long to help out. As Tomi did, he also expresses his concern about Noriko's future. He says that Noriko should forget about Shōji and consider marrying somebody, adding that he feels so bad about her still remaining single. For the first time, Noriko apologetically expresses her true feelings to her father-in-law, the feelings that she refrained from revealing to Tomi:

> NORIKO: There are days when I don't think of him at all. . . . Then sometimes I feel that I just cannot go on like this. Some-times at night I lie and wonder what will become of me if I stay this way. The days pass and nothing happens. I feel a kind of impatience. My heart seems to be waiting—for something. Oh, yes, I'm selfish.
> SHUKICHI: You are not.
> NORIKO: Yes, I am. But I couldn't tell Mother this.
> SHUKICHI: That's all right. You are a truly good woman. An honest woman.
> NORIKO: Not at all.[17]

The recurrent verbal expression, "You are a truly good woman," articulates both Tomi and Shūkichi's feelings about Noriko, and this conversation shows us that Shūkichi means it in the deepest possible sense. Ozu does not tell us *why* this empathy is possible since as a storyteller he is more interested in telling us *what* his reaction to Noriko's confession is. However, judging from the film's progressive action, we can easily deduce that Shūkichi's empathy stems from a life steeped in the empirical knowledge that one cannot reenact the past in the present, that one must accede to the progression of time.

Shūkichi goes to the Buddhist altar and takes out a woman's watch from one of the drawers, which belonged to his late wife. He offers it to Noriko as a memento, saying that Tomi would be happy to see her daughter-in-law using it. Shūkichi adds: "I'm really concerned about you. I want you to be happy—I really mean it." Thereupon, unexpectedly Noriko bursts into tears. Ozu shows her face covered with her hands, in a close-up (not a large one). Ozu does not explain the reason for Noriko's sudden emotional outburst; he merely presents it as a fact. It is another of those rare occasions in which Ozu resorts to a close-up to dramatize an individual character's emotional climax. From the development of the father–daughter-in-law relationship, we can easily surmise that this single close-up constitutes the moment of crystallization of family solidarity; the affection, which has been submerged between Shūkichi and Noriko, finally surges to the fore. Shūkichi says: "It's strange. . . . You have been kinder to us than our own children. . . . Thank you. . . ." In spite of the monotone of his voice, his gratitude is directly transmitted to Noriko's sensitive heart. The scene ends with a medium shot of Noriko trying to suppress her tears.

This outburst of Noriko's emotion leads to the final coda of the film, during which we recapitulate Shūkichi's and Noriko's acceptance of life. Here, as earlier stated, Ozu does not try to oppose and resolve the three different ways of coming to accept the dissolution of the family. The final coda also presents a fine example of Ozu's geographic transition. It opens with shots of an elementary school building. We hear children singing inside. It is Kyōko's classroom. She takes a look at her watch, and a close-up of her face expresses a sudden realization. As soon as she runs to the window and looks down at the train running beneath it, we learn the reason for the insertion of this close-up: Kyōko has recalled that the train with Noriko aboard will pass by very shortly. Now the camera shifts to the running train, and then cuts to its interior. From Noriko's line of sight, Ozu presents a succession of shots of the mountains of Onomichi, indicating her close affinity with Tomi's survivors who remain there. Noriko then puts her watch, the memento, to her ear and falls into a reverie. So far Ozu has frequently introduced the clock and the watch. For example, more than twice he cut to the clock at the station when their children saw Shūkichi and Tomi off.

These images are a clear index of the flux of time, to which human beings are subject. The memento, reinforced by a close-up of the wheels of the train, implies that Noriko cannot revive the past except in memory and that she must leave the past for the future, letting time pass of its own accord.

As the scene shifts to the Hirayama house, Ozu recapitulates familiar commonplaces of everyday life. Shūkichi fans himself, looking out to the distant sea. The next-door neighbor speaks to him. All this "connects" Shūkichi with his new condition: he is alone. Ozu manages these repetitions so deftly that we, the audience, *feel* what we have seen: Shūkichi's solitude and his resigned acceptance of his wife's death.

It is also at this moment that we realize how Ozu's characters have grown. Those members of the Hirayama family who are insensitive to the others' feelings remain as flat characters. On the other hand, the sensitive ones, Shūkichi, Noriko, and Kyōko, have glimpsed a cosmic law—*mujō*. Futhermore, the youngest child (Kyōko), whose perspective has been so inflexible, has also acquired a kind of tolerance, with which she can view the self-centered attitudes of her brothers and sister. Ozu does not present these psychological transformations dynamically, but suggests or implies them. However, the alert viewer intuitively knows and feels them.

Now Ozu takes us to the conclusion of the film. He presents a point-of-view shot of a tiny ship gliding on a distant inlet. Then, he cuts to the profile of Shūkichi still watching the sea. The ship gradually leaves the inlet with rows of houses on both sides for the open sea. The last shot presents the ship as a tiny point on the inlet, while we hear the whistle on the sound track. In this final shot Ozu expresses the world view that is implicit in the film, "a still-life view which connotes Oneness."[18] In the complete fusion of the man-made object and nature the universal law manifests itself: in the reservoir of the fertile life force, human transactions comprise only a single segment like this tiny boat on the vast stretch of the ocean.

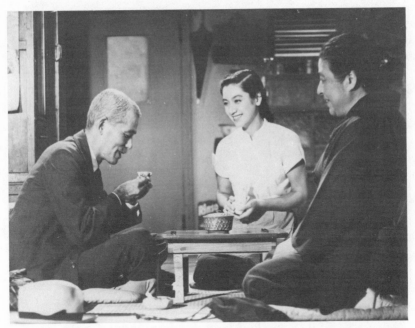

Tokyo Story (1953). Tomi (Chieko Higashiyama), Noriko (Setsuko Hara), and Shūkichi (Chishū Ryū).

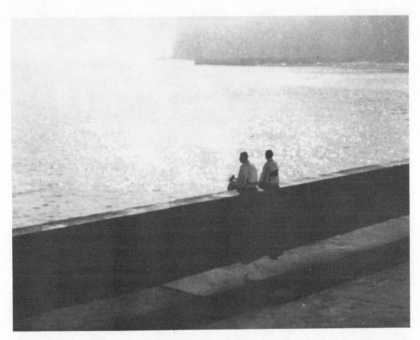

Tokyo Story (1953). Shūkichi (Chishū Ryū) and Tomi (Chieko Higashiyama) at a hot spring resort.

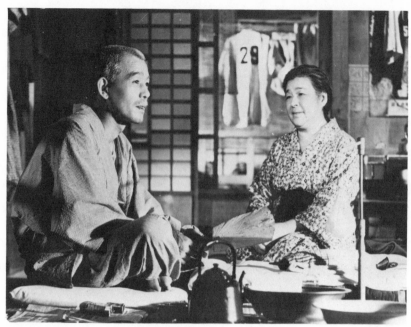

Tokyo Story (1953). Shūkichi (Chishū Ryū) and Tomi (Chieko Higashi-yama).

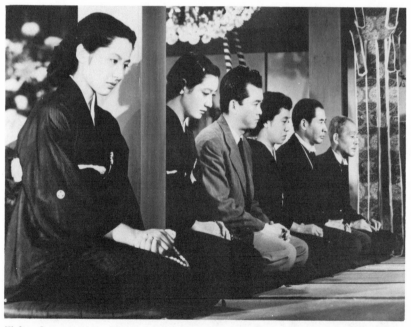

Tokyo Story (1953). Shūkichi (Chishū Ryū), Kōichi (Sō Yamamura), Shige (Haruko Sugimura), Keizō (Shirō Ōsaka), Noriko (Setsuko Hara), and Kyōko (Kyōko Kagawa) at Tomi's funeral.

NOTES

1. Donald Richie, *Ozu: His Life and Films* (Berkeley: University of California Press, 1974), p. xi.

2. Ibid., p. 9.

3. Ibid., pp. 8–9.

4. Ibid., pp. 3–4.

5. Donald Richie's article, "Yasujiro Ozu: The Syntax of His Films," is a comprehensive study of Ozu's basic cinematic techniques employed in his representative works. See *Film Quarterly* 18 (Winter 1963–64):11–16.

6. "Ozu Yasujirō Ron," [On Yasujiro Ozu] in *Sengo Eiga no Shuppatsu: Gendai Nihon Eigaron Taikei* [Departures in Post-War Japanese Cinema: A Collection of Essays on Contemporary Japanese Cinema] (Tokyo: Tōkisha, 1971), 1:203.

7. Donald Richie, *Japanese Cinema: Film Style and National Character* (Garden City, N.Y.: Doubleday Anchor, 1971), pp. ix–xx.

8. Yasujirō Ozu, *"Tokyo Story,"* trans. Donald Richie and Eric Klestadt, *Contemporary Japanese Literature*, ed. Howard Hibbett (New York: Alfred A. Knopf, 1977), p. 191.

9. Noël Burch, *To the Distant Observer: Form and Meaning in the Japanese Cinema* (Berkeley: University of California Press, 1979), pp. 175–76.

10. Ibid., p. 176.

11. Paul Schrader argues the importance of a stasis, an expression of "a frozen view of life which does not resolve the disparity but transcends it." According to Schrader, the progressive degree of disparity, which Ozu's characters experience, leads into a decisive action such as weeping, and this decisive action finally leads to Ozu's presentation of stasis, an expression of the inner unity of every phenomenon, an expression of something unified, permanent, transcendent. It is rather unclear whether this stasis expresses the status which Ozu's character can achieve or the status that simply remains transcendent. See *Transcendental Style in Film: Ozu, Bresson, Dryer* (Berkeley: University of California Press, 1972), pp. 49–53.

12. Ozu, *"Tokyo Story,"* pp. 218–19.

13. Ibid., p. 225

14. Tadao Satō, *Ozu Yasujirō no Geijutsu* [The Art of Yasujiro Ozu] (Tokyo: Asahi Shinbunsha, 1971), p. 286.

15. Ibid., pp. 287–89.

16. Ozu, *"Tokyo Story,"* p. 235.

17. Ibid., p. 236.

18. Schrader, *Transcendental Style in Film*, p. 49. Schrader claims that in Ozu's films, "the image of stasis is represented by the final coda, a still-life view which connotes Oneness." If we follow Schrader's argument, the final shot of the tiny ship on the inlet can be called the stasis because of a harmony existing between the ship and the sea.

Part 7
THE RHETORIC OF FILM

11
Kinoshita and the Gift of Tears:
Twenty-four Eyes

Since his directorial debut with *The Blossoming Port* [Hanasaku Minato] in 1943, the same year Kurosawa directed his first film, Kinoshita has made over forty films. In *Japanese Cinema*, Donald Richie points to Kinoshita's views on traditionalism as the thematic basis that controls the vast corpus of his works. Richie claims that although in his earlier films such as *Broken Drum* [Yabure Daiko, 1949], *Carmen Comes Come* [Karumen Kokyō ni Kaeru, 1951], and *Carmen's True Love* [Karumen Junjōsu, 1952], Kinoshita mocked "the traditional, particularly the family system,"[1] he moved to a defense of traditionalism in such films as *Times of Joy and Sorrow* [Yorokobi mo Kanashimi mo Ikutoshitsuki, 1957] and *The Ballad of Naruyama* [Naruyamabushi-kō, 1958]. Richie's approach offers a keen insight into the internal structure of Kinoshita's films. However, these films can also be meaningfully analyzed in terms of their external structure; Kinoshita knows exactly how to manipulate the viewers' rhetorical stance, that is, their responses to the individual characters' feelings and choices of action.

From this perspective, we can roughly divide Kinoshita's films into two categories: the satiric genre, to which *Broken Drum*, *Carmen Comes Home*, and *Carmen's True Love* belong; and the lyrical genre, to which such representative works as *Times of Joy and Sorrow*, *Twenty-four Eyes* [Nijūshi no Hitomi, 1954] and *You Were Like a Wild Chrysanthemum* [Nogiku no Gotoki Kimi Nariki, 1955] belong. *A Japanese Tragedy* [Nihon no Higeki, 1953], which is generally considered to be the most controversial Kinoshita film, fits into both categories.

The satirical genre, as defined by a number of literary critics, presupposes the audience's complete detachment, from which stance the director either attacks or mocks a set of values represented by a character. Kinoshita's satirical mode is related to Horatian satire; together with the individual characters, who assert nontraditionalism, we laugh good-naturedly at the other characters' obstinate adherence to the traditional way of life. On the other hand, the lyrical genre presupposes audience-character identification: an inside view, thanks to which the audience partakes of the situation with characters, and shares in it. The viewer in the lyrical genre can see the character's world as an extension of his own because of universal qualities inherent in both worlds. Kinoshita is renowned more for his evocation of the lyrical than the satirical mode. *Twenty-four Eyes* (1954) is generally acknowledged to be a paramount example of the typical Kinoshita lyricism and also to be one of the most "lachrymose" postwar Japanese films.[2] Kinoshita knows precisely when he can make the Japanese audience sob and cry.

Western viewers may have to be reminded of the historical background of a film like *Twenty-four Eyes*, if the intentions of its director are to be understood. Kinoshita made this film nine years after Japan's defeat in World War II and three years after the end of the Allied Occupation. This defeat had been the most traumatic experience in living memory for most Japanese, representing as it did the climax of a process of dehumanization, and especially individual sacrifice for collective goals that were later repudiated as being unworthy. By the time this film was made, Japanese audiences had had time to reflect on Japan's involvement in the war—and to reencounter the nation's experience in a manner that Western audiences may not understand. The nature of the Japanese response and Kinoshita's management of it in *Twenty-four eyes* may need some explaining, lest Western audiences see in the film a kind of emotional overkill—mere soap opera, where the Japanese (who have either the experiential or indirect knowledge of the war) find genuine emotional cultural involvement in tragic events.

First, it will be useful to explain the nature of Kinoshita's lyricism as revealed in this film. In most cases, he intends to guide us toward an identification with the protagonist Ōishi and/or with her pupils. But this characteristic of the lyrical genre at times is set aside in favor of a rigorously "outside" exposure to characters. While sympathetically observing their plight, we are nonetheless required to take a detached view in order to get beyond the individual/particular to some broader implication suggested by the director.

The director evokes lyricism in *Twenty-four Eyes* in basically three ways. First, he presents a set of individual characters, who are very much like us in their responses to everyday life. Ōishi, an elementary school teacher, is such a character. She is a delicate, yet spiritually strong Japanese woman, who confronts many stages of hardship caused by the war. We impose our sense of values upon the values that she has, and we view her predicament, often thinking that if we were in her position, we would act as she does. Ōishi's pupils, twelve innocent children, have built very strong emotional ties with her; we watch their lives fatally altered by external circumstances. Their world is not corrupted, and thus is easily accessible to us. We feel no generation gap, but move easily into the children's minds to become one with them.

Second, throughout the film, especially in scenes of emotional intensity, Kinoshita uses popular children's songs associated with certain sentiments as a background. For example, "Furusato" [Home Town], which is a leitmotif of the film, incites in Japanese audiences a nostalgia for their hometown. "Aogeba Tōtoshi" [Farewell Song], which is traditionally sung at graduation ceremonies, brings the audience sweet memories of elementary school, prompting them to share with the twelve schoolchildren both their gratitude for Ōishi and their sorrow over their separation from her.

Finally, the smooth rhythmic continuity of the entire drama makes it very easy to take the inside view. Into the main plot concerning Ōishi's relationship with the twelve children, Kinoshita weaves variations on contrasting moods—joy and sorrow, emotional climax and anticlimax. These moods naturally correspond to the ups and downs of Ōishi and her students' lives. Thus, we are kept from indulging in one particular mode of feeling for so long as to revolt against our identification with the individual characters; we are spared feeling that we have enough of this or that sentiment.

Concerning Kinoshita's "drama of rhythmic continuity," a Japanese film critic, Naoki Togawa, states:

> The drama of rhythmic continuity means the progression of the film's action wherein one scene, one cut, one gesture or one dialogue presupposes the following scene, cut, gesture or dialogue respectively. The sorrowful and despondent scene is followed by the light, joyful scene, and the character's slow gesture reflecting his despondency is succeeded by his quick, vivid gesture of running. And a sweet cheerful episode results in a sad episode. This abrupt transition also constitutes the elements of drama of rhythmic continuity.[3]

Into this lyricism, which is made possible by these three means and which prevails throughout the film, Kinoshita sprinkles periods of detachment, the outside view. This rhetorical tension, a key to our substantial reading of the film, becomes predominant in its latter half. As the individual characters begin to be affected by the trauma of war, and we are shown concrete evidence of its effect and their consequent choices of action, we become more pensive and start questioning their attitudes. Thus, despite the strong lyricism, this intellectual burden keeps us from identifying with any one character because we are more eager to judge the film's content from a much wider perspective than that of any one character.

Moreover, Kinoshita is not a great stylist. He really does not resort to sophisticated camera work to manipulate audience perspective. His method is direct. He relies on standard techniques for his desired effect: frequent use of close-ups and point-of-view shots and timely use of a dolly shot. He also lets his characters verbally display their feelings.

The basic plot of the drama of *Twenty-four Eyes* follows the life of the elementary school teacher, Ōishi, on the island of Shōdoshima in the Inland Sea. The film covers the period from 1929 to 1946 (a year after Japan's surrender to the Allied forces) and can be divided into four sections by subtitles.

The first section concentrates on Ōishi's first assignment to a branch school, which results in the solidarity between her and her twelve pupils. Covering only a part of 1929, this section is pervaded by a rather happy and humorous mood occasionally interrupted by sadness and sentimentality.

The second section, beginning five years after the first one ends, presents Ōishi's marriage and the excursion of the schoolchildren, now sixth graders. The happy mood, which was established in the first section, is now more and more often threatened by sorrowful, serious moods growing out of Ōishi's negative experiences.

The third section takes us to the tumultuous period of Japan's imperialist expansion marked by the China Incident (1937), the Tripartite Pact (1940), and finally World War II. We witness the hitherto relatively peaceful, happy lives of the villagers now becoming clouded by the war and the happy mood relapses into a despondent one.

The last section begins in April 1946. We encounter Ōishi now in her forties going back to teaching again after she has lost both her husband and her youngest child. Feelings of resignation prevail in this section, interspersed with nostalgic feelings for the past and a gleam of hope for the future. It is in both the third and the last sections that we, departing from our identification with the individual characters, are most frequently forced into detachment.

We now examine the film section-by-section in order to illustrate how Kinoshita controls our rhetorical stance. The opening sequence contains two elements that set up the initial mood which is appropriate for our emotional involvement. One is an arrangement of the tune, "Aogeba Tōtoshi" [Farewell Song], which opens the film. This song, as earlier explained, is tied to Japanese feelings of separation and deep gratitude for their teachers, and evokes an extremely sentimental and nostalgic mood. The other element is the geographic setting for the drama, a small village, whose idyllic quality also elicits a rich response from Japanese viewers. Kinoshita moves from the general to the particular in introducing the village. First, we see the Inland Sea with a small boat and a sightseeing ship on it. Then Shōdoshima, the second largest island in the sea, is captured. The shot of the island is quickly taken over by shots of stonecutters and pilgrims. Then, the small village, the location of Ōishi's elementary school, is introduced: a bus is running and women are talking. Japanese viewers spontaneously associate the island with the peaceful, rustic place blessed with the warm weather suitable for the cultivation of olives. We are easily drawn into a nostalgic yearning for nature unspoiled by civilization.

Now the subtitle forces us into our nostalgic affinity with the past in place and time: "If we can call one decade a span of the old time, this story takes us two spans back. . . . The 4th of April in 1929. Elementary school pupils attend the branch school at the cape until they become fourth-graders, and then they go to the main school in the village, walking 5 km each day." The nostalgia, initially established, is once more reenforced by another song, "Furusato" [Home Town]. This song accompanies scenes of separation throughout the film. Thus, the following scene shows a group of schoolchildren running toward their female teacher, who is going to leave the school to marry. The camera cuts to the children's sorrowful faces, and we sense a familylike solidarity between children and teacher in this community. This is where Kinoshita takes full advantage of the emotive quality of the song "Home Town," which explores an adult's recollection of his hometown where he spent a happy childhood. The song thus generates in viewers nostalgic yearning for their hometowns still untainted by progress.

This frankly sentimental mood is challenged by a counterpointed noise, the metallic jingle of bicycle bells accompanying the slow

melody of "Home Town." It is in this transitional state of our
feelings that Kinoshita introduces the protagonist, Ōishi. A young
woman in Western dress passes, riding a bicycle. The children
think that she must be Ōishi, their new teacher. Here, we see an
emotional distance between Ōishi on the one hand and the children
and their parents on the other. The children's initial response is
that she is too modern for this conservative village. Some of their
old-fashioned parents are revolted by the idea of a woman who is
not only attired in Western dress, but is riding a bicycle as well.
Correspondingly, we become objective witnesses to both parties,
instead of letting ourselves be drawn into the world of either; judging by what little the director has offered us, we are not sure
whether we accept Ōishi's world or the children's as an extension of
our own.

However, as the film progresses, the twelve children become
more initmate with Ōishi and a mutual affection develops between
them. Accordingly, without any hesitation we find ourselves
gradually entering the world shared by Ōishi and the children.
This identification takes place for the first time when she lines up
her twelve pupils and says: "From today you are going to be my
pupils and to study hard. Please line up straight. Where are your
eyes looking? Look straight, all right?" Doing as they are told,
the innocent schoolchildren look seriously straight ahead. The teacher
also tells them to say yes clearly. Instead of the expected authoritar-
ian figure, however, she turns out to be friendly to the pupils,
calling them by their nicknames. The twelve children become more
relaxed and comfortable with her. Her democratic attitude as an
elementary school teacher, though disapproved of by some conservative villagers, is acceptable to us, because thinking we would
act like her in her place, we quite easily take the inside view of her
world. In the subsequent scene, we see the proprietress of a haber-
dashery shop talking to two villagers: she complains about Ōishi's
calling the pupils by their nicknames and about her comment that
one of the pupils is cute. With this criticism we become even more
sympathetic toward Ōishi because we share the same value system
with her and rally to her defense.

In the following scene between Ōishi and her mother at their
home, we become even more involved with Ōishi. Through her
mother's words we learn that the bicycle is a necessary form of
transportation for Ōishi who rides it to commute four miles a day,
and that she has had to buy the bicycle on installment. We also
learn that Ōishi's Western black suit is made from her mother's old

kimono. We fully acknowledge that she is just like us and hope that the villagers will soon come to understand her situation. As Ōishi goes over the calligraphy exercises done by her pupils, Kinoshita presents repeated crosscuts between each student's name on the calligraphy paper and Ōishi's face shown in close-up. The director prompts our sympathy for the world shared by the children and the teacher through a conventional means: a combination of a close-up and a song. The background song now is "Nanatsu no Ko" [Seven Baby Crows], which is about a mother crow proudly cooing about her baby crows in her mountain nest. The song, another leitmotif, which expresses Ōishi's affection for her small pupils, strengthens our affinity for her. This feeling acquires a poignant quality—close to tears, in fact, when we hear Ōishi saying: "When I first stood on the platform in the classroom, those small children were tense, exposed to the group life at the elementary school for the first time. I found those twenty-four eyes so cute and thought that I wouldn't contaminate eyes." During the conversation between Ōishi and her mother, we also learn that the children's community is so poor that they, small as they are, have to baby-sit for their little brothers and sisters, or help their parents to hull wheat and to pull fishing nets in on the beach. When Ōishi says that she does not mind commuting to the school rain or shine to educate these poor children, we admire her courage and devotion and can easily share her value system.

Our empathy for Ōishi still continues. The subtitle now signals another interval of time: six months after Ōishi's first encounter with the twelve children. We see teacher and pupils singing "Awate Dokoya" [A Hasty Barber], which reinforces the happy mood they share together. This happy mood, however, is suddenly disrupted when Ōishi stumbles and falls, because of a trap that several fourth-graders have laid for her as a joke. Unaware of what has happened to Ōishi, some of her own pupils start giggling over her fall while others stare in surprise. But as soon as they realize that she has sprained her ankle and cannot get up, the students all fall silent. On the sound track we again hear the leitmotif song, "Nanatsu no Ko" [Seven Baby Crows]. It reminds us of the teacher's almost maternal relationship with the twelve pupils that has been formed for the last six months. When Sanae, one of the twelve students, sees the tears coming from the teacher's closed eyes, she bursts into tears. The other students follow suit. Our natural response is to feel despondent, just as Ōishi and her pupils do.

After this scene, another mode of emotional "identification" de-

velops in a comic interlude. The male teacher, who substitutes for
Ōishi in music class, clumsily conducts the pupils' chorus. Since he
is far from being a musician, the children recite musical notes
intead of a song. The first-graders all look bored, and the substitute
teacher looks irritated. He then orders them to sing "The Prover,"
while he listens. Though the children start singing the song, the
boys whisper: "We cannot sing such a sissy song." The situation is
so amusing that instead of joining either party, we can look at them
and laugh together with the director, the center of the controlling
consciousness.

Soon our detachment breaks down when we begin to realize that
Ōishi's absence is a serious problem for these twelve children.
They all miss her terribly, wondering when she will be back at
school. They climb a hill from which they can see a pine tree near
her house on the other side of the island. Our emotional involvement with the children is made possible through the particular
camera work and a song. Kinoshita uses the dolly shot, which
incites our emotional identification. While the children walk from
the left to the right of the screen, the camera slowly follows them.
When they stop at the top of the hill, it stops on them. When the
children reach the top, Kinoshita uses a point-of-view shot of the
pine tree. This single shot is effective in conveying the children's
feelings; the house is remote but they yearn to see her. On the
sound track we hear "Furusato" [Home Town], the recurrent leitmotif evoking the children's close tie with their small village, which
will eventually be threatened by the war. A series of long shots,
which Kinoshita uses to present the children's movement, also emphasizes their closeness to their surroundings.

While they are watching the pine, the children's desire to go to
see Ōishi becomes stronger, and they finally decide to sneak out of
their houses after lunch. These children do not realize how great a
distance separates Ōishi's house and their village, but we know this
through Kinoshita's earlier point-of-view shot. While the children
discuss their plan, Kinoshita's camera approaches the one-scene,
one-shot method, encouraging us to be attentive to these little boys
and girls' affinity with their teacher and taking us right inside their
minds.

The following day, the children vigorously start their trip. this
time, another song, "Oborozukiyo" [A Night with the Misty
Moon], is heard on the sound track. This song, which describes a
spring dusk glowing over a mustard field tinged with yellow, corresponds to the peaceful mood of the village still untouched by the

threat of war. We also affirm a sense of the children's oneness with their environment.

The lapse of time is expressed through crosscutting to the children's houses where their parents are worried about their whereabouts. The scene cuts back to the children, this time walking along a mountain path, their enthusiasm and energy completely gone. The shift in their feelings becomes evident; accordingly, our feelings shift also. The thread of Misako's *zori* (straw sandals) is now torn, and so is that of Takeichi. Kotoe, who did not eat lunch, starts crying. The others also start crying. Toward the end of their journey, Kinoshita resorts to extreme long shots of the children walking along the country road. This time the long shots serve to evoke their isolation and helplessness in an unfamiliar environment. At the same time the recurrent leitmotif, "Nanatsu no Ko" [Seven Baby Crows], as it merges with the children's crying on the sound track, creates the typical Kinoshita lyricism, making our entry into these pupils' minds natural and irresistible.

Subsequently, Kinoshita relies upon a standard cinematic technique to finalize our empathy with the children: a close-up. First, he presents a long shot of the children walking in tears. Then the camera gradually tracks up to them to single out one boy in a close-up as a token of the twelve children in hunger and distress. The camera follows him to a dissolve, adding a softer sentiment to the scene than a regular cut could have. After the dissolve, we see again a long shot of the twelve children dragging their feet on the road. When a bus passes them, they see Ōishi in it. The despondent, melancholy mood, which has been sustained for some time, suddenly changes into exhilaration. The children all shout, and Ōishi steps out of the bus. As the children circle around her and start crying again, we unhesitantly share this transition of the mood and now feel their relief and the delight of the teacher and her pupils. Another dissolve expresses another lapse of time while adding a soft texture to the film. It yields to a series of shots of the children at Ōishi's house; they are vigorously satisfying their appetites, eating the noodles prepared by her mother. We continue to take the inside view of both the children and Ōishi. We feel like the affectionate teacher, who is content to see the children enjoying their meal. At the same time, nostalgically going back to our childhood, we put ourselves in the place of these children, who are enjoying a home-cooked meal near the teacher they love.

After this scene, a photograph of Ōishi and her pupils standing against the ocean is taken by a professional photographer. This

picture becomes fixed in our mind as an index of the unbreakable
bond between them. It is a simple yet effective means of eliciting a
sentimental response. As a result of this incident, the children's
parents, whose conservative attitude is not attuned to Ōishi's modern attitude, become more amicable toward her; they sincerely
show their gratitude for Ōishi and her mother's hospitality to their
children by bringing her gifts of rice, wheat, and sesame. Just as
Ōishi does, we feel delighted with this apparent change in the
parents' feelings and attitude. Consequently, we experience mild
resentment and disappointment with Ōishi, when, encouraged by a
member of the education board and persuaded by her mother, she
submits to their desire for her to move to the main campus. We
wonder why Ōishi, who has been so devoted to her pupils, must
leave them to accept a new position. The inconvenience of commuting to the distant branch school on a bicycle strikes us as inci-
dental; our values cannot accept such an opportunistic attitude on
the part of Ōishi.

This mild antagonism of ours gradually eases during the next
scene in Ōishi's demonstration of warm feelings for her pupils.
When she has told the children at school that she will be transferred
to the main school, the camera focuses on the children for a long
time, evoking tension as an objectification of their feelings. The
music on the sound track, "Annie Laurie," adds a sentimental
touch to the film's texture. The children are all silent with tears in
their eyes. When the camera cuts to Ōishi, we also see tears in her
eyes. As soon as one child starts crying aloud and snuggles against
her, the others follow suit. When they see her off as she gets into a
small boat, the children sing the song, "Nanatsu no Ko" [Seven
Baby Crows]. The camera moves from one child to another, inviting our identification with each. Our affinity for the children
deepens when Kinoshita introduces a point-of-view shot: Ōishi's
boat gradually disappearing into the distance. The long duration of
this shot also strengthens our affinity.

The second section creates a radical change in our responses to
the individual characters. The relatively complacent feelings,
which we have shared with Ōishi and her pupils, begin to merge
with emotional tension as Japan's jingoistic mood starts to affect the
residents of even this small island. The subtitle says:

> The ocean and mountains are just the same as they were five years
> ago. However, in the past five years, the Manchurian Incident and the
> Shanghai Incident have occurred, and the depression has set in. Not

knowing what would await them in the near future, the children have grown, experiencing their own joy and sorrow.

The children, sixth graders now, are singing, "Kōjō no Tsuki" [The Moon Over the Ruined Castle] on the boat rowed by Masashi, one of Ōishi's pupils. This song immediately evokes in the Japanese audience the ephemeral quality of all earthly phenomena. We naturally wonder about the vicissitudes of life these children are to confront as they grow older.

The scene cuts to a harbor. The children encounter a party of formally dressed adults headed by the principal of their school; the party is going to greet Ōishi's bridegroom coming from a ship. The song with the light rhythm, "Minato" [Harbor], describing a number of ships tossed by golden waves, enhances a sense of joyous expectation. Together with the children we initially experience the excitement of waiting and together with them also we laugh heartily when they mistake a chubby middle-aged man with a mustache for the bridegroom.

The happy mood established at the beginning of this section suddenly collapses into a despondent one after Matsue, who has been watching the bridegroom's party, is suddenly told by a villager to hurry home. Kinoshita then cuts to Matsue's dingy house where her mother has just given birth to a baby. In order to draw our attention to the poverty of the family, Kinoshita uses a one-scene, one-shot method to present Matsue's family; the mother is in bed with the newborn baby, while Matsue prepares lunch for both her father and herself. The father hurriedly eats a bowl of rice. Matsue wants a lunch box with a lily pattern on it since all her classmates have such a lunch box. Matsue is ashamed to take her lunch box to school. Kinoshita strongly engages our sympathy, again by a standard filmic code: a close-up of Matsue's old wicker lunch box, a concrete image of the poverty of her family.

A new lunch box, though trivial to most girls, becomes an obsession with Matsue. When the scene moves to the school, she smilingly approaches Ōishi, now married, to tell the teacher that her mother gave birth to a baby. Matsue does not fail to add that her mother will now buy her the lunch box she has long wanted. Our feelings toward this little girl are strong, but judging from what little Kinoshita has shown us about her family, we suspect that her dream may not be fulfilled.

After this scene, the film lapses into a more tense and tragic situation. We are taken back to Matsue's house and see her father wiping tears and Matsue holding the baby in the presence of Ōishi. Matsue's mother has died. Her father tells Ōishi that he cannot send Matsue to school because she has to stay at home to take care of the baby. He also adds that the baby would be better off if it were not alive, that nothing good will come of it, raised in such a poor household. Matsue does not look pleased when Ōishi gives her a lunch box with a lily pattern, which she has bought for her. Our hearts go out to the father and daughter; however, we are denied identification with them. We cannot be the father, whose extreme poverty blinds him to the respect of his baby's life; neither can we assume the child's point of view, since Matsue is too small to grasp the entire situation, especially what is going on in her father's mind. We thus see this domestic tragedy from the perspective of Ōishi, who though an outsider, is capable of both sympathy and empathy. Becoming one with her, we want to encourage poor Matsue as Ōishi does, saying: "You have to help your father. I am always thinking of you at school. You are such a nice girl. . . ." We accept poverty as a universal problem and at the same time we feel pity for individuals swept away by forces beyond their control.

From this tense domestic scene Kinoshita cuts to the school and shows that political forces are affecting even the small village school. Ōishi learns that a colleague, Mr. Kataoka, has been investigated by the police who suspect that he might be a Communist. She also learns that one of Mr. Kataoka's ex-classmates is an anti-war activist, and that the police are looking for *Kusanomi* [Seeds of Grass], a collection of creative writing by the ex-classmate's pupils as a proof of Mr. Kataoka's conversion to communism. Ōishi protests that she has seen the journal and that she even read some of the writing to her pupils because she thought it good. Hearing this, the principal orders her to get rid of her copy of this journal. There ensues a shot of Ōishi looking at the journal in flames in a brazier. To emphasize the sense of suppression of individual freedom (epitomized by the seizure of *Kusanomi*), Kinoshita again introduces a clear-cut cinematic code: Stephen Foster's funeral song on the sound track.

When the scene changes to the classroom, we see Ōishi questioning her pupils. She asks how many of them read the newspaper at home and if they know the meaning of "the reds," Communists, capitalists, and the like. Later, we see Ōishi being reprimanded by the principal for teaching her pupils the taboo subject under the current political system. Through their ensuing conversation, Kinoshita engages us in "intellectual" detachment for the first time.

Ōishi responds: "My pupils heard about Mr. Kataoka and *Kusanomi*, and they wanted to know why he had been questioned by the police." The principal says: "You should have pretended ignorance. We live in a time when we really must watch what we say. You have to be careful. How on earth did you dare to tell your pupils about the proletariat and the capitalist?" We, the Japanese audience, admire Ōishi's courage in insisting on leading her pupils to the truth despite the dangers. While sympathizing with her situation, however, we rhetorically do not allow ourselves to identify with her. We are more anxious to judge opposing points of view from a much wider perspective, becoming more and more aware of the extent of the sociopolitical forces influencing the individual's life as well as his outlook on life.

Our objective detachment, momentarily assured, again dissolves into our emotional involvement, when Ōishi learns from one of her pupils that poor Matsue has been taken away from the island by a strange woman. Through the mouth of this innocent informant, Kinoshita tells us all that is necessary for us to know about Matsue's fate: "Matsue clung to the pillar at the entrance to the garden and cried that she would not go. Her father first cajoled, but finally pushed her back and beat her head." Hearing this, Ōishi puts a handkerchief to her mouth and starts sobbing. We now enter into her mind, and together with her we cry (or sob) over Matsue's plight. Our identification with Ōishi still continues, while an extreme long shot of her walking in the rain conveys her despondency.

Following Matsue's departure, the film again presents variations in rhythm; it makes a joyous turn and shifts back to a sad one. It is now October, the time for the school excursion. We see Ōishi smilingly surrounded by her pupils aboard a ship bound for Shikoku. Each pupil tells her how he or she has got money for the trip. Jinta says: "Others have scrambled for money. But my father's business has been so good that he has bought me a new school uniform for the excursion. . . ." When Jinta starts showing off his clothes we notice that they are too big for him, as is his new pair of shoes. Along with the teacher and her pupils, we laugh at his outfit. Temporarily transported back to our school days, we enjoy each moment of the school excursion with the same pleasure we experienced in our own school days. A sightseeing boat approaches their ship and Ōishi keeps looking at it and smiling. We realize that the approaching ship is her husband's. Against the background music of "Home Sweet Home" played by the band aboard the sightseeing ship, the two ships pass each other. This is a happy moment and we smile with her, accepting her joy and affection for her husband and pupils as an extension of our normal feelings.

Once again, however, joy relapses into sadness. When they arrive at Takamatsu, Ōishi feels ill. She and a female colleague decide to eat a bowl of hot noodles at a nearby eating place so that she will feel better. There Ōishi finds Matsue, who, though she was supposed to be in Ōsaka, is now working here as a waitress. Neither Ōishi nor Matsue has much to say to the other, and the proprietress of the place keeps talking to Ōishi and her colleague. We do not have to be told how Ōishi and Matsue feel. Having watched their relationship develop since Matsue was a first-grader, we understand their feelings at this reunion. Thus, when Kinoshita shows us both Matsue's and Ōishi's backs, we can take an inside view without being prompted visually.

The following scene is one of the most tearful scenes of the film and has a carefully calculated Kinoshita flavor. Matsue runs through a small alley and is just about to come out to a thoroughfare to see Ōishi and her colleague walking back to the harbor. All of a sudden, she stops and hides herself in the alley as she sees her former classmates pass by talking to Ōishi. Again we hear the familiar "Nanatsu no Ko" (Seven Baby Crows) on the sound track, reminding us of a close relationship between the teacher and her pupils. In order to make us cry, Kinoshita does not have to show Matsue's face in tears. Instead, he presents a back-shot of her sobbing and gazing at the ship leaving the harbor with her former classmates and teacher aboard. Kinoshita employs a dolly shot when Matsue walks from the right to the left of the screen as the ship glides in the same direction. The camera follows her until the ship is out of sight. This method effectively demonstrates Matsue's loss of ties with her former classmates. With handkerchiefs clasped in our hands, we proceed to the following scene.

As the action progresses, we become more fully aware of the socioeconomic forces that are affecting the children's fates. Together with Ōishi we become discouraged by, and resigned to, the individual's inability to fight against the larger-than-life forces of history. After the pleasant excursion, the pupils are now back in the classroom; they must write a composition with the title, "My Goal in the Future." Here, Kinoshita again appeals to our sentimentality by presenting another tragic event. All of a sudden, Fujiko starts crying, and confides in the teacher that her father is bankrupt and that her family will soon have to vacate their house.

Fujiko also adds how much she wanted to go on a school excursion with her classmates. Conceptually we accept Ōishi's naturalistic view when she starts explaining to Fujiko in simple terms that individuals are victims of forces beyond their control. At the same time emotionally we share her despondency and feel like crying as she says to her pupil: "Your suffering is not your fault nor your parents'. You must be strong. This is all that I can say. When you feel like crying, please come to see me any time. You and I will cry together."

From now on, Kinoshita varies our mood response less frequently as the film takes us relentlessly along the path of history. Now that the fates of Ōishi and her pupils are firmly entrenched in our hearts, we are asked to step back and consider the place of mere individuals in the context of a very dark period in human history.

Accordingly, the next scene shows Ōishi and Kotoe alone in the classroom. Kotoe confesses to her teacher that she has to quit school after she completes the sixth grade since she must cook for her family while her mother is at work fishing and her younger sister is still at school. Kotoe also adds that she has written in her composition how she wishes she had been born a boy because she feels sorry for her mother. Ōishi also learns from this pupil that she will be apprenticed to a seamstress after her little sister completes the sixth grade. During their conversation, Kinoshita uses a one-scene, one-shot method, inviting us to take the inside view of the two, specifically of their mutual trust. However, as soon as Ōishi asks Kotoe if she will marry after working in Ōsaka, and the little pupil answers affirmatively with her smiling face, the one-scene, one-shot method yields to crosscutting between the two, emphasizing two distinctly different views on woman's role: marriage as her medium for security, and her independence through a meaningful profession. Ōishi does not look pleased with Kotoe's answer that she will follow in her mother's footsteps and marry after completing her service as a seamstress, though she takes pity on her mother's misery. The succeeding two shots—a close-up of Ōishi's face and a shot of the heavy shower outside—effectively convey Ōishi's anger over social inequity and her inability to console Kotoe. We silently acknowledge that if we were a teacher like her, we would feel the same way.

In the next scene, a few days later, we see Ōishi speaking to three boys in the playground. To these pupils, who all want to be soldiers, she says: "Why do you all want to be soldiers?" One of them asks Ōishi if she does not like soldiers, and she answers that she prefers fishermen and rice dealers. Later, she reveals her honest feelings to one of her female pupils: "My boy pupils are saying that they want to become soldiers, but I am afraid to let them die." Considering the historical setting of the film, a period when the Japanese people were being subjected to indoctrination by a fanatically militaristic government, we admire Ōishi's honesty even as we fear the consequences of her candor.

As expected, the following scene presents another confrontation between Ōishi and the principal. While emotionally siding with her, we become objective observers of both parties as we are again anxious to examine opposing views from a wider vantage point. Ōishi claims that as a teacher she tries to be honest with her pupils and to tell them the truth. The principal objects that in the middle of a national movement toward armament she should not have the audacity to tell the boys not to be soldiers. Ōishi protests that she simply respects the life of each pupil. Her superior insists on the prevailing view: that she should keep silent; that the teacher's duty is to educate pupils so that they can serve their country. We recognize the validity of what the principal is saying, given the temper of the times and the tragic turn of events that history has made familiar to us. Yet emotionally we are closer to Ōishi's view as we want to accept her individualistic attitude as more universal and less literally insular.

After this incident, another melodramatic scene, the graduation ceremony, occurs, awakening our nostalgia for our school days and the sadness at parting from them. Ōishi's ten pupils (Matsue and Fujiko have left the island) are now going to graduate. Against the music of "Aogeba Tōtoshi" [Farewell Song] evoking sadness, the camera pans up to Ōishi and then moves from one child's face to another. Each is bathed in tears, which some brush away. The camera pauses for some time on Ōishi weeping, and then travels along the cherry blossoms nearby to capture an entire tree in a close-up. This traditional Japanese image effectively creates again a feeling of impermanence. The music, the symbol of cherry blossoms, and the close-ups of teacher and pupils, all in harmonious order, help to present the feelings shared by them and to provide us with a smooth entry into their minds.

The following scene captures Ōishi expressing her true feelings to her husband. She says that now a teacher is allowed to communicate with her pupils only through the government-designated textbooks and that the teacher-pupil relationship is perfunctory. She is also distressed over the fact that all her male pupils want to become soldiers. She adds that her husband should also quit his job as a sailor so that they both can become farmers. Her husband replies that he cannot agree with her. Our affectionate concern for Ōishi is undiminshed, even as we know too much of history to take her idea of running away seriously. We, however, deny ourselves identification with her because we are more oriented to viewing the effects of war upon individuals in their totality rather than viewing them from one particular character's perspective.

In the third section of the film, we are confronted with the more immediate effects of the war upon individual lives, as the subtitle indicates: "The ocean and the mountains are the same as yesterday. But the villagers' lives have been swept by large historical events such as the China Incident and the Tripartite Pact. . . . Eight years have passed." Here Kinoshita invites us to vacillate between involvement and detachment. Since the effects of the war are presented from the viewpoint of Ōishi, we must take the inside view to experience them as her felt reality, but at the same time we must assume the outside view to grasp them in their totality. In other words, we are right into history and out of it, as well.

This section opens with a shot of Kotoe's place. Kotoe is now pale and thin, lying in bed in the storage shed of her house, entirely isolated from the rest of her family. Mellow sentimentalism, naturally culture-bound and designed to make the audience cry, is evoked through two unsophisticated elements. One is a close-up of the photograph of the twelve children. The other is a familiar subject matter shared by many sentimental Japanese novels: a poor girl becomes a victim of tuberculosis after she sacrifices herself to the needs of her family. Ōishi comes to visit Kotoe. Using a point-of-view shot (from Ōishi's perspective), Kinoshita shows us all that is necessary for us to know in order to emphathize with Kotoe: her isolation and the poor condition of the shed. The ensuing close-up of the photograph, the only decoration in the place, reminds us of the close affinity between the teacher and the pupils that has withstood the progression of time. The war has also had a great effect upon Ōishi. We are surprised to see how tired and old she looks.

After Kotoe relates her misfortunes, she and Ōishi sob together. Kinoshita obviously invites the audience to share in these tears as the camera cuts to the photograph once more pausing in a close-up of each face in succession as the leitmotif song, "Nanatsu no Ko" [Seven Baby Crows], plays in the background.

As the film progresses, we are more and more exposed to the effects of the war. We see many villagers leaving the island to join the service, seen off by their families, relatives, and friends, who shout "Banzai!" (Hurray!). At Ōishi's house we see her husband holding a conscription notice in his hand and facing his mother-in-law. For the first time we learn that Ōishi now has three children—two boys and a girl. We now fully acknowledge her feelings about the war; she does not feel the duty and obligation that the nation wants to impose upon her. Instead, she is full of her own emotional responses to the war. During this period of Japanese history, whenever a Japanese received a conscription notice, it was customary for his family to celebrate his entry into service by serving him sake. Ōishi, however, refuses to do this, protesting that there is no cause for celebration. Though we are very sympathetic toward her genuinely expressed private feelings, our view of the value system is torn between individualism and collectivism. We begin to wonder how we would have behaved if we had been Japanese mothers and wives living in this war period, which required of individual citizens complete patriotism. We thus say to ourselves: "Could we have been patriotic enough to cancel our private feelings for the so-called common good and to send our husbands and children to war without fuss; or could we have been more personally courageous and expressed our individual sorrow and indignation openly just as Ōishi did?" We become more pensive and try to reach a reasonable conclusion concerning these two opposing value systems, thus denying ourselves identification with Ōishi.

This philosophical question becomes more immediate as World War II looms closer in the film. The subtitle intervenes: "The last four years have witnessed an increase in tombs of soldiers, who participated in the war." There ensues a shot of a group of teenagers, who volunteered for air force service, walking down the pier to leave the island. We spot Daikichi, Ōishi's eldest son, among those who see the group off. When the camera cuts back to Ōishi's house, her husband is absent and her mother is confined to bed. Ōishi is absorbed in expressing her antiwar attitudes to Daikichi. She is now middle-aged, and her face and appearance clearly show creeping age and fatigue in contrast to the youth and vigor we saw in her earlier. Daikichi says: "I wish I were a middle-school student so that I could volunteer for service." His mother responds: "Do you want to die in the war so badly? You don't mind your mother living in tears every day in spite of the fact that I am devoted to you body and soul, do you?"

Then, their argument ensues:

DAIKICHI: Then, you cannot possibly be like Yasukuni's mother.

ŌISHI:	Do you think that she is such a great mother? I'm just your mother. Daikichi, I simply want you to be an ordinary human being, an ordinary person who respects his life.
DAIKICHI:	No mother says things like that.
ŌISHI:	They just don't express their true feelings in words. But they think that way.
DAIKICHI:	Even my schoolteachers don't say what you said.
ŌISHI:	Since I was honest, I quit teaching.
DAIKICHI:	You're a coward.
ŌISHI:	I don't care even if I am called a coward. I don't have to be respected by anybody. I simply care for you, Namiki and Yazu.

Now that we have fully heard Ōishi's stance regarding the war, we empathize with her maternal feelings for the welfare of her children. Again, however, despite its superficially simple quality, the conversation between Ōishi and her son lays bare a deeper philosophical issue: "What would have been the right ethical attitude to assume if we had been put in her place?" Because of the intellectual strain aroused by this question, we still remain empathetic observers of her plight, kept from identifying with her. Hence, our emotional response will be that we understand how she feels as a wife whose husband is fighting in the war and a mother of the three children whose existence will be her sole support in case of her husband's death in action. But what is the real courage under the circumstances?—to encourage her children to serve for their country by hiding her true emotions, just as shown by many a mother during the war, or to reveal her true feelings to her children by teaching them the value of human life?

With this rhetorical tension we proceed to the scenes of Ōishi's domestic unhappiness. Kinoshita introduces these scenes with a careful calculation to draw tears from us—especially from the female audience. We see Ōishi running in the rain without an umbrella to Daikichi standing on the pier to tell him that his father has been killed in action. As Ōishi disappears in the rain, holding Daikichi, we now shift from the empathetic observers of her plight and enter into her mind to share her sorrow as a universal human being. No close-up of her face is necessary nor is the verbal presentation of her sorrow. We feel her desperate effort not to cry.

This sympathetic identification remains predominant throughout the rest of the film. A later scene depicts another tragic incident in Ōishi's life, which takes place immediately after the end of the war. We witness Ōishi, in an almost deranged state, carrying her little daughter to the doctor's office, after she has fallen from a tree.

When the camera cuts to the interior of the office, we find this little daughter, Yazu, lying dead on the operating table. After the doctor leaves the office, Ōishi starts crying and her little boys follow suit. Taking the inside view of her situation, we, the viewers, also sob, as she sobs: "Poor Yazu, I don't blame you for having climbed a persimmon tree to satisfy your hunger. You are still holding such an unripe persimmon in your hand. You climbed the tree because you were hungry and eager to get some persimmons. . . ."

The last section of the film begins with the subtitle: "April the 4th, a year after the end of War." We are deeply touched when we see Ōishi looking so old for her age and attired in the shabby kimonolike ensemble required during the war, rather than the black suit she used to wear. She has gone back to teaching to support her family and commutes daily by boat rather than by bicycle. At the same time, we understand the lapse of time, during which she has experienced so many things that drastically affected her life. In the classroom, we see that she is in charge of her former pupils' little sisters and children. As she calls the roll, a tear rolls down on her face. The turmoil and unrest in her mind seems to have subsided and what we feel together with her is the silent resignation, with which she will face the remainder of her life.

This acceptance of the flux of time in recognizing the mutability of human affairs *(mujō)* is a traditional Japanese attitude of life, and becomes increasingly predominant toward the end of the film. Ōishi offers a bunch of flowers at the graves of her ex-pupils, who were killed in the war. She recalls the past in front of one pupil's grave, saying: "Takeichi, you used to say that you would rather be a soldier than a rice-dealer. But now, see what you became!" We are captured by a poignant sense of *mujō* just as much as she is. At the same time, urged by our desire to see this individual experience of hers from a historical perspective and thus to derive a deeper implication from this scene, we step aside from her world momentarily. As humanists we encounter the sense of futility and waste implicit in the war. Realizing that so many young men sacrificed their lives to collective duty, we begin to wonder if this was really worthwhile.

The final scene brings Ōishi and six of her ex-pupils—two men and four women—together. These pupils, now grown up, hold a reunion party for her at the restaurant run by Masuno, one of the six. We find Ōishi really old and inclined to be tearful. In direct confrontation with the passage of time, we recapitulate what each person has encountered for the past seventeen years. Together with Ōishi and her six former students, we rejoice over their reunion and share their memories of the past. Kinoshita employs two particular images to intensify our nostalgia for the past and thus to enhance our sympathy for the participants in the reunion. One is a new bicycle that her ex-pupils have bought so that she will not have to depend on the boat to commute to school. This new bicycle takes us back to the days of Ōishi's youth when she used to ride her bicycle, full of vigor and zest for education. Becoming one with the teacher, whose face is full of wrinkles and whose hair is streaked with gray, we deeply appreciate the tender caring for their teacher that these pupils have never lost in spite of the drastic changes in their lives.

The other image is the photograph of Ōishi and her twelve pupils, which has recurred throughout the film. To guarantee another surge of sobbing from the audience, Kinoshita introduces one of the ex-pupils, Sonkichi, as a victim of war. He was blinded in action and is now apprenticed to a masseur. He turns his face toward the picture. Prior to this scene, Kinoshita presents a medium shot of the picture, reintroducing "Nanatsu no Ko" [Seven Baby Crows] to pave our way into Sonkichi's mind. In response to Sanae's remark that he *can* really see the photograph, Sonkichi says: "I can see it. In the center is Mrs. Ōishi. In front of Takeichi, Jinta and I are standing. . . ." We identify with Sonkichi and share his plight. When the camera cuts to Ōishi looking at him and wiping her tears, we also become one with her and feel her pity for this blind youth. Just like her, we cannot stop our tears.

The subsequent scene of Ōishi's two sons throwing stones at the ocean is taken over by the scene of Ōishi riding her bicycle in the rain, then getting off to push it up a hill. On the sound track we hear "Aogeba Tōtoshi" [Farewell Song] once more. Now we are brought strongly face to face with the feelings of *mujō*, which keeps the traditional Japanese in accord with the passage of time, never resenting or trying to fight against fate. We really do not feel any indignation against the injustice done by war to these survivors—Ōishi, her fatherless children, and the blind Sonkichi. Instead, we encounter the feelings of quiescence, which lead the individual characters to accept things as they are. It is in *mujō* that we spectators, Ōishi, and her ex-pupils are finally united together.[4]

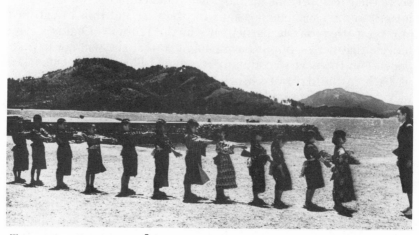

Twenty-four Eyes (1954). Ōishi (Hideko Takamine) and her pupils.

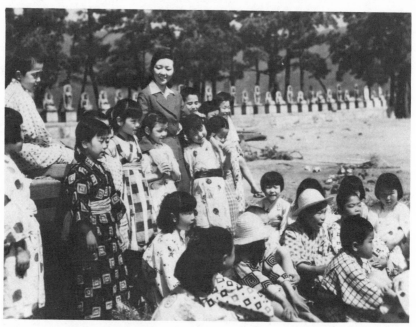

Twenty-four Eyes (1954). Ōishi (Hideko Takamine) and her pupils.

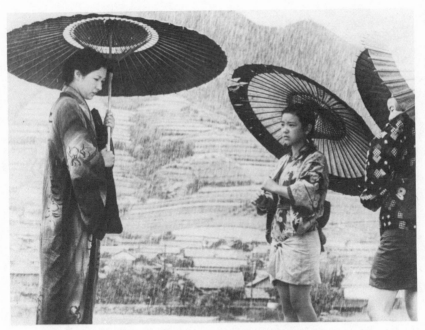

Twenty-four Eyes (1954). Ōishi (Hideko Takamine) with her children.

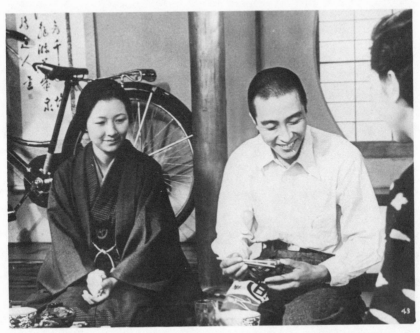

Twenty-four Eyes (1954). Ōishi (Hideko Takamine) reunited with her ex-pupil (Takahiro Tamura).

NOTES

1. Donald Richie, *Japanese Cinema: Film Style and National Character* (Garden City, N.Y.: Doubleday Anchor, 1971), p. 97.

2. Both Satō and Nanbu attribute this film's melodramatic quality to two aspects; first, released during the postwar period when Japanese audiences still remembered their own experience in the war vividly, the film exploring individuals' confrontation with the war had an immediate impact upon these spectators. Second, the film, which portrayed the individual characters' endurance and sustained love, instead of ugly phases of the war, against the background of the lovely landscape, incited their tears. See *Nihon Eiga Hyakusen* [One Hundred Selections of Japanese Cinema] (Tokyo: Akita Shoten, 1973), p. 141.

3. Naoki Togawa, "Kinoshita Keisuke: Sono Nihonteki Shishitsu" [Keisuke Kinoshita: His Japanese Quality] in *Kinoshita Keisuke Kantoku Tokushū* [Special Issue on Keisuke Kinoshita] (Tokyo: Film Center of the Tokyo National Museum of Modern Arts, 1972), p. 6.

4. Satō claims that *Twenty-four Eyes* is rather sentimental in that it depicts a simple lamentable fact that "good-natured people bitterly suffered from evil political forces encroaching on their lives." He also emphasizes that Kinoshita's *Carmen's Pure Love* and *A Japanese Tragedy* are more dynamic in exploring Japan's tragedy and her people's. However, it seems that Kinoshita does not expect us to interpret *Twenty-four Eyes* as a political genre film but that he wants us to see it as a lyric genre film. See *Nihon Eiga Shisōshi* [The History of Intellectual Currents in Japanese Cinema] (Tokyo: Sanichi Shobō, 1970), p. 267.

12
Viewer's View of *Odd Obsession*

Kon Ichikawa's *Odd Obsession* [Kagi, 1959] is based on the novel by Junichirō Tanizaki that shocked Japanese readers by dealing frankly with sex. The film, like the novel, does more than that. It takes as the object of its satire a respectable middle-aged couple in contemporary Japan and shows what happens to them when they determine to rejuvenate themselves through sex rather than resign themselves to advancing age in the traditional Japanese manner.

Since the film, like its book, is heavily satirical, the director must arrange for a certain amount of detachment from the viewer. The nature and function of satire demands that much. What is fascinating about Ichikawa's directing is the enrichment that he brings to the satirical mode by manipulating the audience's point of view in several ways.

First and most obviously, Ichikawa gives us the novelist's characters: people whose values are strikingly at variance with the accepted norm. Thus, we are confronted with a disparity tested in action. Ichikawa improves on the novel by giving the servant Hana a more important place in the action, and a more troubling rhetorical presence as well. She is not directly involved in the ugly sex game played by the four major characters, but functions as a detached observer on the scene—with an important fillip of irony to add at the end.

Ichikawa's use of irony, being both visual and verbal, is somewhat more complex than in the novel. The film constantly directs our attention to important and revealing differences between what the characters say and do and how, deep down, they feel and respond. Thus, obsession may be shown as odd because of the satirical disparity, yet it still conveys a sense of psychological insight, as irony suggests more truth than can be presented "face-on."

Finally, there is Ichikawa's finesse with camera techniques. His

style in *Odd Obsession* is all the more interesting because he uses
standard devices like wide-angle shots, crosscutting, and camera
placement both to position his subject with great insight and suggestive power and more importantly, to distance the audience, involving us, through a carefully detached point of view, in a
coherent vision of this other world in which these people scheme
and betray one another so oddly.

At the very outset, we are given the central problem of the film in
beautifully ironic clinical fashion. The young intern, Kimura, delineates the physical symptoms that a man exhibits at various stages
of aging: "Our physical deterioration begins at the age of ten when
our eyes lose their resilience. At twenty, our auditory sense begins
to decline. At forty, our palate is no longer sensitive to subtle
tastes. At sixty, our olfactory sense deteriorates. . . ."

This seems reasonable enough, so as Kimura continues, we are
lulled into acceptance, tempted to see in him the reliable physi-
cian's prognosis, the reliable plain truth told by a detached observer. No wonder we are even tempted, as viewers, to identify
with him. Suddenly, however, we notice a subtle mocking, ironic
tone as he points a finger directly at the audience, saying: "No one
can escape growing old. Not even you, spectators, who are going to
watch this film."

Suddenly, we are truly detached, filled with doubts about the
value of Kimura's argument, and his purpose in turning it against
us. And when he appears as a character in the drama, we have
every reason to remember the distance between him and us.

Thus, Ichikawa dramatically poses the central problem of his
film: "How is a middle-aged couple to cope with the fact of aging?"
Implicit in that problem are two conflicting choices: submission to
the flux of time, or a perverse denial of it.

Odd Obsession deals with the perverse second choice made by
Kenmotsu and Ikuko, husband and wife, who try to use sex as a
weapon against old age. It is, ironically, a neat family drama, since
Kimura is to be married to Toshiko, the daughter of Kenmotsu and
Ikuko. This young couple will be drawn to their destruction
through compliance with the dangerous sexual strategy of their
elders.

Thus, we have Kenmotsu, a collector of antiques, refusing to
accept old age himself. He deliberately puts Kimura in a way to
make advances to his wife in order to arouse his own jealousy.
Kenmotsu reasons that jealousy, being sexually stimulating, will

help him to recover the physical gratification that he enjoyed with Ikuko in their youth—and, therefore, to recover youth itself. Kenmotsu is asking far more than mere gratification, however; he wants to reverse the very passage of time.

Similarly, after a period of reticence, Ikuko abandons the social mask of wifely modesty, and sees in Kimura the husband who no longer exists: the vigorous youthful mate who can give her the utmost in sexual pleasure. By putting herself in her daughter's place, she too is trying to recapture the past by indulging in present sex. As odd as anything in this drama is the fact that Toshiko connives in her fiancé's affair with her own mother.

Such is the complex state of human affairs with which Ichikawa has to work in this film. He offers us a variety of points of view to work with as we detach ourselves from this conflict of characters and values in order to reach for the sense of wholeness that satirical insight offers us.[1]

We meet the protagonist Kenmotsu after the intern's speech on aging. He is getting a hormone injection in the doctor's office. The claustrophobic dimness of the room suggests the patient's fears. The subsequent close-ups of the reading on a pressure gauge and a wickedly sharp hypodermic articulate his fears. We start to share Kenmotsu's fear of death and we begin to identify with him. Then we see that Kenmotsu is insisting on this treatment, in spite of the doctor's advice to the contrary, and we discover that his visits to the hospital are made on the sly. We detach, and gradually we shift from sympathetic observers to objective, amused spectators. A universal human problem has narrowed to the perspective of individual choice. Kenmotsu's obsession with sex is too singular, as it were, to take us in.

Kenmotsu emerges from the hospital and boards a trolley. The squeaking of the trolley suggests the erratic beat of an ailing heart. Kenmotsu gets off, and freezes on the film. This is a jolt. Does Ichikawa mean to suggest that this man's heart has stopped? Or is this a visual emphasis only, enhancing our expectation of some scene to follow in a crosscut? We are caught between the subjective state of sympathy for Kenmotsu and the objective sense of a film in progress. We encounter a mode of transition back and forth between the elements of a complicated action.

The freeze frame does indeed lead to a crosscut. The rhetorical tension dissolves as this time we see Ikuko in the doctor's office. Ichikawa has made use of a moment of transition to confuse us momentarily so that he can educate our caution in the face of these events. The alert viewer will be aware of being positioned for detachment.

Ikuko's behavior seems perfectly normal, modest, and wifely. Hesitantly, she converses with the doctor, Kimura's boss, about sex. In response to a question, she says in all apparent innocence: "My husband says that he is very creative about sex." But then, as she leaves the doctor, her eyes meet those of Kimura, the intern who lectured us at the beginning of the film. There is something pointed about the display of indifference in Ikuko's eyes, something in the way Ichikawa has shown her actions and her motives. Again, we detach from a character whose "universal" has become a "particular." Just which particular, we do not know yet. Naturally, we suspect that behind the respectable wifely social mask lies a latent unruly sexuality that will lead to something. Ikuko goes home in a taxi. When she steps out of it, she freezes on the film. This time we are sure that detachment and caution are going to pay off.

As expected, Ichikawa crosscuts to the same doctor's office. This time we meet Toshiko standing in the doorway, asking Kimura why he has failed to show up for a date. Her cynical tone surprises us. This is not what we normally expect from a Japanese girl of her age. Then, too, she conveys a certain furtiveness to which we do not quite know how to respond. All we have to go on is a feeling of mild repulsion—just enough to detach us from her.

Now we are "in place." The scene is set for our first outside view of all four characters together. They are seated round a table in the living room of Kenmotsu's house, where Kimura has come for a visit. In place of close-ups and other point-of-view shots, Ichikawa gives us a number of wide-angle frames, as if to avoid establishing any definite point of view on this scene. We get the message: these are four *dramatis personae*. It is up to us to synthesize their complex interactions and to make use of appropriate abstractions in order to connect with the coherent vision of the film. In other words, Ichikawa has made his position clear. He presents these particulars and puts them through their motions; it is up to the viewer to make them yield to universals.

From this point on, the film presents two major movements. The first concerns Kenmotsu's pursuit of rejuvenation through sex, focusing on the extent of its absurdity and its ironically fatal consequence. The second movement concerns Ikuko's progress in the same direction. Once she hesitates, and then chooses passion over reason, with consequences that are equally ironic and fatal.

The movements begin together, as we see Kenmotsu arranging to leave his intoxicated wife alone in the living room with Kimura. He spies on them, hoping to feed his libido on jealousy. Meantime, Toshiko is spying on her father spying on her mother left alone with her fiancé. We detach with a vengeance from this dangerous game, and prepare to witness the consequences. But we must witness actively. In lieu of merely adopting one or the other character's view of events, and the values that they confirm or contradict, we take in all the evidence and synthesize it. A complex film like this gives us a new sense of seeing.

Next we see Kenmotsu arranging more blatant kinds of compromising situations to feed his fantasy-fed desire. He takes nude photographs of Ikuko and asks Kimura to develop them for him. More directly yet, he intoxicates Ikuko purposely, so that Kimura will have to help him carry her unconscious from the bathtub to her bedroom. Afterwards, we see Kenmotsu valiantly passionate over his unconscious wife and we realize how absurd he is, how his determination to deny the fact of aging is downright comical, how this would-be monster of depravity is just a pathetic, silly old man.

This major movement of the film completes itself in two striking scenes that complement one another with deft irony. The first shows Kenmotsu taking nude pictures of Ikuko lying on the bed. Ichikawa employs an extremely wide shot horizontally across the screen, using Kenmotsu to cover Ikuko's shame, as it were. There is a sense of the director's camera surreptitiously photographing Kenmotsu surreptitiously photographing his nude wife. We laugh. There is something undeniably comical about Kenmotsu seen this way, blocking our view of the indecent picture he is trying to snap, amateurishly enough, in bad light, trembling with insufficient lust. We laugh because Kenmotsu, quite objectively, is ridiculous. We are detached, mocking observers. We have him now.

Or so we think. The other striking scene confronts us with one of the paramount ironies of the film. Kenmotsu is making love to Ikuko. Suddenly, he shakes and collapses over her. We are amused by this naked display of the middle-aged man's orgasm. But we are mistaken. The next scene shows that Kenmotsu, in fact, has had a stroke. But this amuses too, as we are that surprised by this reversal of our hasty optimism. The particular lustful enterprise of the perverse old Kenmotsu is universalized right under our noses. When Kenmotsu dies later, we are a little too lighthearted even to pity him. There is too much "rightness" in what has happened. Our final position on Kenmotsu's death is detached; we are lighthearted observers studying man's folly, not Juvenalian satirists out to remedy it.

The second major movement of the film deals with the other three characters. Here, repulsion rather than amusement is the key response as we see the victims of Kenmotsu's obsession turn into obsessive schemers.

Our first impressions of Ikuko are unpleasant ones. Ichikawa presents us with a symbol of her uneasy, suppressed sexuality: a deformed female cat she sees on returning home from the doctor's office. We see in a close-up of the cat a resemblance of Ikuko's face. Here we see the very animal sexuality she wants to hide. We calmly watch her throw the cat out. We sense in this a conscious reaction, a desire to cast out an urge that Ikuko sees as perverse at this stage.

Later, after she has fainted in the bath and Kenmotsu has made love to her, Ikuko tells him innocently that she does not remember what happened. We do not believe her already at this point. We detect a perfect awareness and enjoyment of the sex that came of her husband's game. Kenmotsu mentions that Ikuko's upbringing in a temple has endowed her with virtuous modesty. He is sincere, while we weigh the irony in his remarks.

Ichikawa develops our sense of the difference between visible action and hidden motive. He is a master of revealing discrepancies in a likeness. He shows us the face of the benign Kannon, Goddess of Mercy. We smile to see how like Ikuko's face it is, because the likeness contradicts itself. Passion, not compassion, is Ikuko's true inner note. We see this in an image of appalling clarity as she stands at the sink cracking ice for her bedridden husband. The look on her face here, like the ice pick in her hand, speaks for a desire to kill the husband whom she is nursing.

Ikuko is so plainly repellent that we are alerted to suspicions that are well borne out by later events. We see her rushing home late from shopping, and we know the value of her excuses. She goes with Kimura and Toshiko to a movie. Afterwards, Toshiko excuses herself, as does Kimura, remembering that he is on duty at the hospital. Yet Toshiko leaves first; and we can be reasonably sure, watching Ikuko and Kimura together, that they will soon be off to bed.

Our sense of Ikuko is complete when we see her giving her future son-in-law a key to the house. She will pursue infidelity under the same roof where her ailing husband is confined to bed. More details are provided by a third party, a nurse. Clearly, we are prepared for the moment when Ikuko intentionally takes off her clothes and tempts her husband to the lust that will lead to his death. We are not amused by Ikuko in that scene. Her deviations from the norm are too extreme. She outrages our sense of "universals" too much, the norm here being behavior suitable to a Japanese woman brought up as a priest's daughter.

As we have seen, Kimura aroused our suspicions at the very outset of the film. And in so many ways, he has shown himself to be remarkably compliant. No wonder we watch his every move, looking for clues that may reveal the name and nature of his feelings for Ikuko and Toshiko. He is, in his way, a model of discretion, yet even his bedside manner betrays him as he examines Ikuko after her swooning in the bath. A number of such touches add up to a sense that Kimura's interest in Ikuko is purely sexual, especially since the mother is prettier than the daughter.

Kimura's relationship with Toshiko is more plainly in view. He shows her the nude pictures of Ikuko that her father has asked him to develop. Toshiko promptly challenges his interest, offering to take her mother's place in the flesh. Ichikawa interrupts the love scene that follows in the proverbial cheap hotel with a view of two trains coupling. This parody of Western cinematic technique is more than a touch of Ichikawa's famous black humor. It places Kimura's interests fairly well. Taking a cue from the visual pun, we can say that he is out to make connections. He mentions Kenmotsu's patronage a number of times, and confesses that his own family is poor, so we can surmise that Kimura plans to marry Toshiko for reasons of gain. In a dramatic monologue after Kenmotsu's death, he says so plainly: "I am so disappointed that the family is now destitute. Ikuko is pretty, but not a money maker. Toshiko is by no means pretty. Why in hell did I get involved with this family?"

Kimura stands fully revealed, and is easily judged: he is a social climber caught in his own trap. No ambiguity attaches to him, and the case is dismissed.

Toshiko's motives in all this are more difficult to judge. As we have seen, she is immediately repellent in a subtle way, yet her behavior puzzles us. She spies on her parents; and indeed, she seems remarkably well informed about their goings-on. Ichikawa also allows us to spy on Toshiko. We see her willingly enter into the sex game that her father has set in motion. She goes so far as to help her mother arrange a tryst with her own fiancé. All this suggests that Toshiko's motive is fairly direct; she wants to get back at her tyrannical father.

There is more to it than that. We see Toshiko later on, testing the effect of the truth first on her father. Sure enough, she gives his jealousy full measure, telling Kenmotsu about Kimura and her mother. But then we see her testing Ikuko as well by implying to her mother that she knows about Ikuko's involvement with Kimura. We realize that Toshiko is a far more dangerous type. Playing the sex game with her own set of rules, she is attempting to destroy both her father and her mother. Any connection that we might have felt with Toshiko is broken; her sardonic pleasure in destruction is too much. It particularizes her once and for all.

The pattern of irony is completed by the servant Hana. In earlier scenes, Ikuko has taunted the old woman for her poor eyesight. Yet Hana is something like a seer, though she articulates no moral judgment. She does effect a judgment, however, when she poisons Kimura, Ikuko, and Toshiko. Vengeance is an elderly maid. What we can make of this is that Hana, like us, has been aware of the goings-on in the house. She is a model of detachment, and yet she adds the final finality to the film. Ichikawa explained the reason in an interview given to Joan Mellen in 1974:

> MELLEN: Why does the servant poison the three surviving people at the end of the film? This aspect of the plot was not in the original novel by Tanizaki.
> ICHIKAWA: I wonder if I can get this across to you in Japanese via an interpreter. I'll try. These three people are representatives of the human without possessing human souls. They are not really human beings. The servant is going to annihilate them because the servant represents the director. I wanted to deny them all.
> MELLEN: Then it is the moral judgment of the director on these three people?
> ICHIKAWA: Yes.[2]

It is one thing for a director to kill off his villains, and quite another to ask us to take that act as a reference point for the moral judgment which we must, as the audience for satire, take as clarified. On the contrary, this motion of the director strikes us as too didactic, too obtrusive an attempt to force us into an identification with Hana or, by extension, with Ichikawa himself.

Thus, we ask ourselves a question: Can he really mean it? Is he really offering us in the interview one twist of irony too many? Certainly, in the final scene there are detachments aplenty. Hana is confessing to premeditated murder. Her eyesight is not to blame for the mix-up of containers, one red and one green; one poison for the rats and one soap for the dishes. Yet the policemen cannot believe it. They have too much common sense, too much bureaucratic and unimaginative experience of human nature to credit the tale that this old lady has to tell. The psychology behind this shocking parody of respectable family life escapes these law-and-order men entirely. They can only conclude that Hana is *non compos mentis*. They give events a stolidly conventional explanation; Ikuko and Toshiko, left impoverished, committed suicide, and the young intern Kimura joined them in sympathy. We smile at this four-square paradox. The case is closed. The dead can rest, respectable in peace. Hana is free to go.

Still, a question lingers: Just whose odd obsession have we been viewing with detachment, anyway? (The Japanese title, *Kagi*, means simply "the key," though it has a sexual connotation in the film). Or was it really that of the four, whose game took over their lives? Or was it Hana, who was obsessed with watching them destroy one another before she decided to destroy them herself? Or was it the police, obsessed with the norms and therefore blind to real human complexity? Or was it some aspect of ourselves, some dangerous bit of *otherness* that the satirist sets up for all to see who have eyes to see?

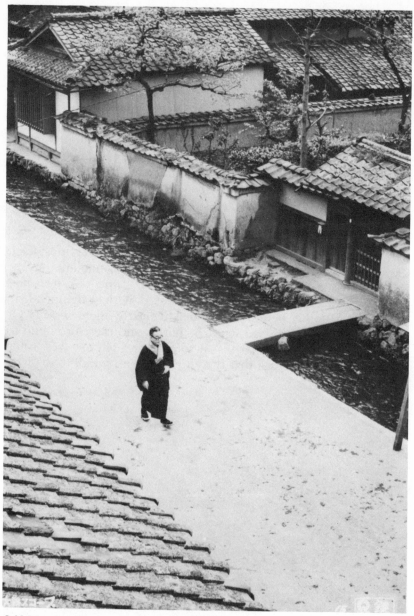

Odd Obsession (1959). Kenmotsu (Ganjirō Nakamura) on his way back from the hospital.

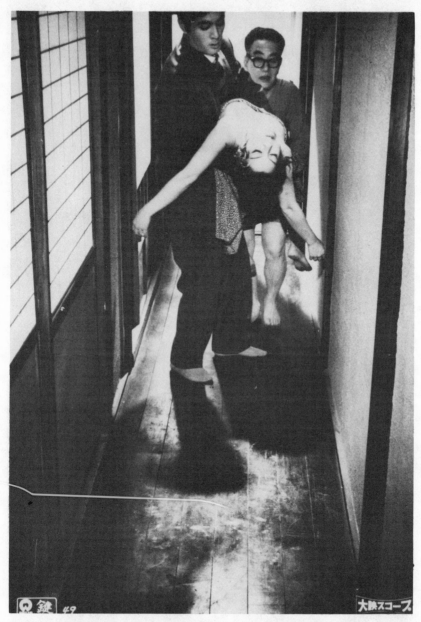

Odd Obsession (1959). The fainting Ikyko (Machiko Kyō) carried by her husband (Ganjirō Nakamura) and Kimura (Tatsuya Nakadai).

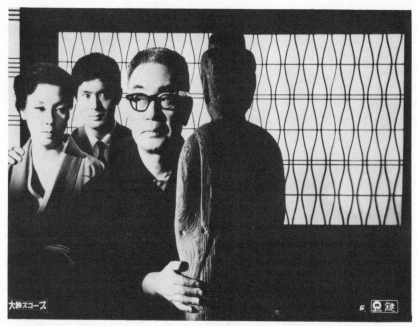

Odd Obsession (1959). Kenmotsu (Ganjirō Nakamura), Kimura (Tatsuya Nakadai), and Ikuko (Machiko Kyō), from right to left.

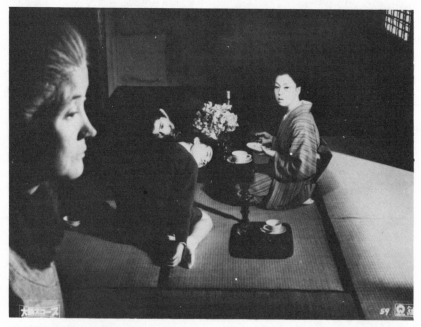

Odd Obsession (1959). The old servant (Tanie Kitabayashi) executing her scheme of poisoning.

NOTES

1. William Cadbury states: "The basic distinction between the outside and the inside view, then, is whether our attention is directed most strongly towards the singularizing attributes or the universalizing problems of a character." "Character and the Mock Heroic in *Barchester Towers*," *Texas Studies in Literature and Language* 5 (1963):569. The article is an excellent explication of the different points of view of the individual characters that the audience must assume in order to achieve a coherent reading of the novel.

2. Joan Mellen, *Voices from the Japanese Cinema* (New York: Liveright, 1975), p. 123.

Conclusion

It is all too well known that no critic can hope to have the last word in any discussion of a work of art. Art is, by definition, more provocative than that. A film critic has to be especially wary of false finality because he or she deals with an art whose immediacy to its audience imposes special conditions. Literary critics have long accustomed us to their task of taking such conditions into account. They show us how authors long dead took readers, long dead as well, into account; and how we must adjust our perspectives accordingly. Literary critics also invite us to add new perspectives, since we are who we are, and since an important test of "great" art is the test of adaptability this way.

A critic is just one member of the audience who studies cinematic art, taking its special conditions into account. Naturally, there will be as many ways to do this as there are critics. In this book, for example, I have tried to show how a few Japanese directors, in a certain few films, have made use of a creative tension between what might be called film-as-presented and film-as-experienced (or film-as-responded-to). The former would refer to the internal structure of the film itself: characters, camera work, themes, and the like. The latter would refer to the external structure: the audience-film relationship. Those same internal elements are designed to reach out and manipulate the audience present and reacting to what is shown on the screen.

The result, as we have seen, can be a challenge to see that there is more to a given film than meets the casual eye. At the risk of overextending our terminology, we might say that the major directors discussed in this book use elaborate rhetorical strategies aimed at persuading viewers to bring two worlds together: a "world out there" in the film-as-presented, and a "world in here" in the film-as-experienced.

The reversal of terms is surprising—certainly the "world in here" should refer to that on the screen—but this reversal speaks for the